Ian Donald
A Memoir

Ian Donald

A Memoir

James Willocks
and
Wallace Barr

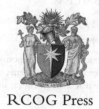

RCOG Press

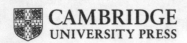

Shaftesbury Road, Cambridge CB2 8EA, United Kingdom

One Liberty Plaza, 20th Floor, New York, NY 10006, USA

477 Williamstown Road, Port Melbourne, VIC 3207, Australia

314–321, 3rd Floor, Plot 3, Splendor Forum, Jasola District Centre, New Delhi – 110025, India

103 Penang Road, #05–06/07, Visioncrest Commercial, Singapore 238467

Cambridge University Press is part of Cambridge University Press & Assessment, a department of the University of Cambridge.

We share the University's mission to contribute to society through the pursuit of education, learning and research at the highest international levels of excellence.

www.cambridge.org
Information on this title: www.cambridge.org/9781904752004

www.rcog.org.uk

Registered charity no. 213280

First published 2004

A catalogue record for this publication is available from the British Library

ISBN   978-1-904-75200-4   Paperback

RCOG Press Editor: Jane Moody

Design: FiSH Books

Contents

Illustrations

Acknowledgements

We gratefully acknowledge the help obtained from the "Sources" listed at the end of the book.

We also have to thank those of our friends and ex-colleagues who contributed anecdotes and reminiscences. In particular, Dr Alistair Miller was of great help in recollecting many of the amusing and sometimes dramatic incidents that occurred along the way.

Mr Alastair Irvine of the Medical Illustration Department of the Royal Hospital for Sick Children was responsible for preparing the photographs and for this we are thankful.

Finally, we most gratefully acknowledge the immense help provided by Margaret Lindsay. As well as putting the whole thing together, she typed it impeccably and prepared it for publication contributing, incidentally, a number of valuable observations and suggestions. It is true to say that, without her help, the book would not have seen the light of day.

Permission has been sought and has been received from copyright holders for all textual material previously published.

James Willocks MD FRCOG FRCP (Glas)

James Willocks died shortly after the completion of this book, a work which all his colleagues thought he was uniquely fitted to write.

He was a registrar with Ian Donald in Glasgow in the late 1950s, the latter working to develop ultrasound as a clinical tool in the face of considerable scepticism. James Willocks was a strong supporter and his contribution was the introduction of fetal cephalometry, which remained for years the only objective way of measuring intrauterine fetal growth.

James Willocks was a natural scholar who brought his learning and sense of humour to all his professional activities: clinical practice, teaching, writing and speaking. His outstanding public speaking brought pleasure to many who did not know him personally.

This book is dedicated, with the greatest affection, to his memory.

AWFM

Preface

To write the life of a great man, as James Boswell wrote at the beginning of his biography of Dr Samuel Johnson, is "a presumptuous task". We do not presume to do this on the basis of comprehensive historical knowledge and wise Olympian judgement, with all details correct and no stone left unturned and we pray the forgiveness of our readers for omissions and inaccuracies scattered throughout this book.

Our object is to provide a personal memoir of one who was our mentor, colleague and friend for more than thirty years and to do this before "Time, like an ever-rolling stream bears us and other contemporaries away – or allows them to descend into amnesia".

We wish we had been like Boswell in keeping the diaries and accurate notes of conversations that make his book a masterpiece. For example, on 31st March 1772, Johnson said to Boswell, "Nobody can write the life of a man but those who have eaten and drunk with him". While this is not entirely true, it encourages us. We did eat and drink with Ian Donald and our aim is to show him as he was. As we go along, we shall ask ourselves, not whether every feature we record was attractive, but whether it was characteristic.

Ian Donald was a vibrant, controversial character who deserves to be remembered for many things in addition to his contributions to ultrasound. In many aspects of his practice he was revolutionary and he was always receptive of new ideas. He was an inspirational teacher, a caring clinician who was adored by his personal patients, and a stimulating and provocative colleague. He endured great suffering with much courage.

He was never in doubt about what was right and wrong in the world and consequently met with much opposition when his views were not politically correct. He was a true "Renaissance Man" of many talents and he was never dull.

But, of course, his greatest contribution was in medical ultrasound. As has been said elsewhere, "If you seek his memorial, look around you – and in every maternity hospital you will see ultrasound in use".

Early Life

Ian Donald was born on 27th December 1910 in Liskeard, Cornwall, the eldest in the family of two sons and two daughters of John Donald, medical practitioner, and his wife, Helen Barron Wilson, concert pianist. John Donald came from a Paisley medical family and his brother Hugh was surgeon to the Royal Alexandra Infirmary. John led rather a peripatetic life, practising in London, Lichfield, Penang, Liskeard and Leicester. He served in the Royal Army Medical Corps during the 1914–18 War.

Helen Barron Wilson met her future husband in Penang, while she was on a concert tour of the Far East.

Ian's early education was at Warriston School, Moffat, and then at Fettes College, Edinburgh, a public school which now has a prime minister among its former pupils. He conceived a lasting dislike of Fettes and later he quoted with approval the remark of a schoolfellow who had survived a Japanese prisoner of war camp and saying "It was just like being at Fettes".

The family then went to live in South Africa, for health reasons. Ian's father had tuberculosis, and was never able to practise in Cape Town. The disease progressed and he died when Ian was only 16 years old. His mother died in the same year. Ian's sister, Dame Alison Munro, records "Ian's character and his powerful influence on his family and those around him emerged at the age of 16. He forcefully led his sisters and his brother in resistance against relatives in the UK who wanted to split the family up. His leadership of the family continued throughout his life".

Ian finished his schooling at the Diocesan College, Rondebosch, and after that graduated with a BA from the University of Capetown in French, English, Greek and music.

During these years he acquired his deep knowledge of literature. The Bible and Shakespeare were second nature to him and quotations constantly illustrated his conversation and his writing. This breadth of his education is in striking contrast to what is on offer to medical students nowadays.

He returned to England in 1931 to study medicine at St Thomas' Hospital Medical School in London. Even as a student he had an original approach to problems and an interest in gadgets. He devised a bladder irrigation machine for women with chronic infections, a sensible idea in the pre-antibiotic era. Unfortunately, on one occasion it burst while in action, drenching a patient and her husband, so that it did not become popular!

Ian graduated in medicine in 1937 and in the same year married the love of his life, Alix. She was also from South Africa and was born in Bloemfontein during the great influenza epidemic at the end of the First World War.

At one stage Ian thought he might become a psychiatrist. However, the story goes that, on sorting through his father's effects, he came across his box of surgical instruments – an indication to him of the direction his studies should take. After a number of junior hospital appointments, war broke out and he joined the Royal Air Force (Medical Branch 1942–46). He was decorated for gallantry for going into a burning bomber, with its bombs still in it, to rescue injured airmen (MBE, military, 1946).

Already he was marked as a man of outstanding qualities.

In London 1946–54

In 1946 Ian was able to come back from his war service to his beloved St Thomas' Hospital, one of the most prestigious of London's historic teaching hospitals.

St Thomas' (named after Thomas à Becket) was founded in the twelfth century. In the early fifteenth century, Lord Mayor Richard Whittington (of "turn again" fame) made "a new chamber of eight beds for young women who had done amiss, in trust of a good amendment". In 1535 it was called by a government official "the bawdy hospital of St Thomas in Southwark", not because of young lady patients but because the master kept a concubine and had sold the church plate. In 1561 unmarried pregnant women were refused admission because the hospital was erected for the relief "of honest persons and not of harlottes". In the virtuous Victorian era, the hospital had emerged from its chequered past and a vast new edifice was built in 1871 on a block principle that was approved by Florence Nightingale, who established in it the Nightingale School of Nursing and thus revolutionised the nursing profession. From then on, St Thomas' nurses were known as "Nightingales". The medical school also opened in 1871.

St Thomas' and its associated Lambeth Hospital and the Chelsea Hospital for Women were busy centres for obstetrics and gynaecology and that was the specialty that Ian chose to follow on his return from the RAF. Then, as now, young doctors in this field were overworked and got very tired, as the following short note to Alix emphasises.

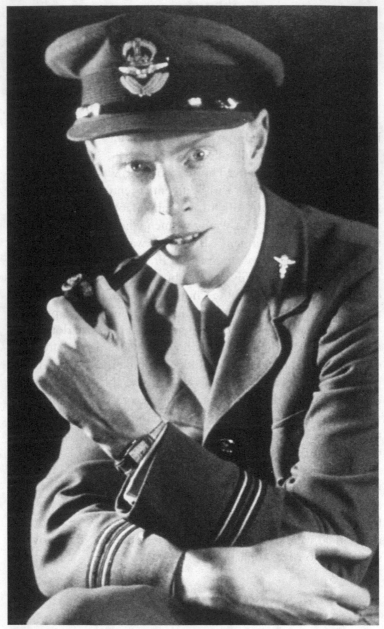

In the RAF

We think that all obstetricians and their spouses can empathise, for they have been through it too.

Ian was distressed and became fascinated by the problems that babies faced passing through the "valley of the shadow of birth" as he called it and later he directed enthusiastic research efforts towards the problem of respiration in the newborn.

In the post-war years the London medical scene was enlivened by many interesting characters. In gynaecology, the outstanding figure was the flamboyant surgeon Victor Bonney (1872–1953), whose main work was done before the War but whose influence persisted. He was appointed gynaecological surgeon to the Middlesex Hospital in 1908. His *Textbook of Operative Gynaecology* was first published in 1911 and was still current for MRCOG students in the 1950s. It contained 611 beautiful line drawings done by himself. In surgery too he was an artist and a master of surgical technique.

In operating theatres all over the world it was possible to recognise by a surgeon's skill with his hands that he had been taught by the master in London. Bonney developed conservative techniques for non-malignant conditions of the uterus and ovaries, such as fibroids and ovarian cysts. With no children of his own (because of surgery which his wife had in youth) he developed these techniques for the relief of infertility. At the same time, he was the greatest exponent in the Western World of radical pelvic surgery for cervical cancer.

Victor Bonney's pupil, Charles Read, a New Zealander who eventually became President of the Royal College of Obstetricians and Gynaecologists, had a great influence on Ian Donald. From Bonney, Read learned not only the technique but the art of surgery. He was one of the most dextrous radical operators of his generation and Ian followed his techniques. Sir Charles Read was a big man, full of energy, who worked and played hard and lived life to the full: such a man was Ian Donald.

Another surgeon Ian used to talk about was Louis Carnac Rivett (1888–1947). He was a rapid and spectacular operator who enjoyed showmanship. He had his opportunity, as gynaecologists from all over the world came to see him work. Again, some of his style probably influenced Ian.

At St Thomas' Hospital, Ian revered James Wyatt (1883–1953) who had been obstetric physician there since the end of the First World War. Wyatt was a first-rate teacher with excellent clinical judgement and a sympathetic nature. A bachelor and bon viveur, Wyatt loved organising social occasions and left a generous bequest to the RCOG – enough money for the Council of the College to hold one dinner annually.

But perhaps the most influential of Ian's teachers at "Tommys" was AJ ("Joe") Wrigley (1902–1983), the inventor of a refined and gentle obstetric instrument, "Wrigley's forceps". He was a down-to-earth Yorkshireman whose motto was "Experience is the best of teachers – but his fees is very heavy".

Ian frequently quoted this motto. Joe Wrigley gained a Gold Medal for his MD thesis in 1928 and in 1936 he was appointed consultant physician in the department of obstetrics. In 1946 he became head of the department, which under his leadership became one of the foremost in London.

Joe Wrigley was "crafty" in the fine old Yorkshire sense of that word. He knew how to keep his patients out of trouble and when trouble struck his reactions were swift and sure. He was a great manipulator in all senses of the word and had a wicked sense of humour. Sometimes he would contrive awkward situations for pompous colleagues so that he could witness their downfall; it was fun to see so many behave in exactly the ways he had predicted. This was a technique that Ian copied and rehearsed before trying it out on visiting dignitaries and external examiners.

The story of Wrigley's forceps is that as the storeman at St Thomas' was tidying up he came across a pair of small obstetric forceps with straight blades – a pattern originally devised by William Smellie in the eighteenth century. Joe immediately saw their value, went to an instrument maker and said, "Put a pelvic curve on these and shorten the handle". His forceps have to be used gently and lightly and this has certainly prevented much damage to baby and mother.

Joe was a great teacher. He was kind and encouraging to all his juniors; he reserved his humorous criticisms for his peers. Ian was undoubtedly a favourite pupil and he enjoyed Joe's company at meetings after he had retired.

In 1947–48, as Ian worked at St Thomas' Hospital, the London medical establishment, like doctors all over the country, was greatly disturbed by the proposed introduction of a National Health Service. The Minister for Health, Aneurin ("Nye") Bevan, an eccentric and uncontrollable star of the Labour Government, was locked in endless stormy negotiations with the British Medical Association, which, jealous of its professional privileges, hated change and abhorred Bevan. On the other side, the Socialist Medical Association demanded "no concessions – a full-time salaried staff, no private beds – the socialist dream, the whole dream and nothing but the dream". But Bevan, despite his maverick tendencies, was a sincere and practical man. No other politician has been so closely in touch with realities of working class life. Many of his ideas for the NHS came from the "medical aid" schemes in South Wales, which the miners had financed and organised themselves. Bevan had the sense to get to know the heads of the Royal Colleges and other influential men. This was achieved through contact with his childhood friend Dan (Sir Daniel) Davies, who enjoyed earning good fees from his well-to-do patients in Wimpole Street and also enjoyed giving free advice to poor people. It was around his hospitable table that Nye Bevan was able to meet, in total privacy, the leaders of the medical profession. Relations changed surprisingly quickly from hostility and suspicion to willingness to cooperate. In the end, the Health Service survived all opposition and became law.

The 1950s and 1960s saw the golden age of the Health Service. It was a time of innovation and idealism when all things seemed possible. Ian was a keen advocate of free treatment, whole-time practice and hospital reform, as he showed convincingly when The Queen Mother's Hospital opened in 1964.

Whether Ian welcomed the introduction of the National Health Service or not we do not know. He was probably too busy to worry about such matters. In 1952 he left St Thomas' Hospital on being appointed Reader at Hammersmith, London.

The British Postgraduate Medical School at Hammersmith Hospital was opened by King George V in 1935, the year of his Silver Jubilee. The hospital, formerly known as the Workhouse Infirmary, was situated next door to Wormwood Scrubs prison. In the economic gloom of the 1930s it is remarkable that it opened at all. In fact, the opening was described as a "glittering gathering".

Sir Austen Chamberlain, brother of Neville and chairman of the governing body told the King that the school was to have three main tasks: the continuing education of general practitioners, the training of specialists and, most important of all, the pursuit of research and the advance of medical knowledge. The King responded with reference to the "happy union of ward and laboratory".

Academic medicine had been slow to develop in London, and Hammersmith's aims of combined clinical teaching and research were ideally suited to Ian, who was an enthusiast for both. During its first seventeen years, Hammersmith benefited from high-quality staff, including James Young and Chassar Moir in obstetrics and gynaecology. It survived the war years when it became a casualty hospital of 400 beds. Not being in Central London it received people who were dug out of bombed buildings and were often found to have crush injuries. Another big problem was jaundice and Sheila Sherlock (aged 28) was in the team that defined the pathology of hepatitis; this was the first step in her career as an outstanding teacher and investigator of liver disease.

The war firmly established the school's reputation for teaching. Many courses were held in all subjects and many Americans and Canadians came to hear a new radical approach to medicine. The post-war years saw the introduction of new antibiotics, the most important influence on the practice of medicine. It was also an era that was to be dominated by new technology. There were biochemical techniques such as flame photometry, paper chromatography, mass spectrometry for the analysis of gases and metabolic balance studies. There were new radiological techniques such as vascular imaging and radioactive isotopes were introduced into clinical investigation. All these had a major impact on the school's researches.

Ian Aird, in charge of surgery, was a stimulating and innovative teacher. He encouraged work on haemodialysis for renal failure and for a pump oxygenator (heart and lung machine) to facilitate open cardiac surgery. The first open heart operation in Britain was performed by WP Clelland in 1954. Bill Clelland became Britain's leading heart surgeon in the 1960s and will reappear later in this narrative. It was an exhilarating era, with a revolution in the intellectual approach to medicine, leaving no established medical belief unchallenged. This was the sort of atmosphere that Ian enjoyed to the full. Hammersmith was a place where there was a fizz of excitement that gave a champagne quality to every day. Professor J McClure Brown was head of obstetrics and gynaecology and his department made important contributions, including early studies of exchange transfusion for haemolytic disease of the newborn and studies of placental function.

When Ian joined in 1952, his earlier publications had given no idea of what was to come; they were 'pot-boilers' on uterine rupture and the aetiology and investigation of vaginal discharge. Now he had the chance to respond to a real challenge – the problem of respiration in the newborn. He measured experimentally the very first breath of life and devised apparatus to help babies breathe when respiration did not get off to a flying start. His work was a forerunner of modern methods in neonatal paediatrics.

In 1954 he gave the Blair Bell lecture at the Royal College of Obstetricians and Gynaecologists on the subject of atelectasis neonatorum. In that same year he developed a patient-cycled respirator, which went by the name of the "pneumotron". He brought this instrument with him to Glasgow and we remember many evil hours spent trying to get it to work.

Because of his interest in machines, Ian was known as "Mad Donald" by some of his London colleagues who caricatured him as a crazy inventor, but senior men had already noted his rare talent and just at a stage when he was considering emigrating to Canada, the Regius Chair of Midwifery at Glasgow became vacant on the retirement of Professor Lennie.

Appointment to the Glasgow Chair

We do not believe that Ian had ever dreamed of working in Glasgow. That "dear green place" was, in the minds of most of the London establishment a dirty, dreary industrial town, peopled by savages. Many London consultants and academics in the 1950s shared the view expressed in the 1770s by Dr Samuel Johnson: "Men bred in the Universities of Scotland cannot be expected to be often decorated with the splendours of ornamental erudition, but they obtain a mediocrity of knowledge, between learning and ignorance, not inadequate to the purposes of common life". Yet Glasgow University was founded in 1451 by Pope Nicolas V (who also founded the Vatican Library) and its constitution was based on that of the Pope's own University of Bologna, the oldest in the world. In Britain only Oxford, Cambridge and St Andrews were its seniors. In the eighteenth century, Glasgow graduates William Smellie and William Hunter laid the foundations of rational and scientific obstetrics. In the nineteenth century, Glasgow Professor Joseph Lister had saved countless lives by his discovery of the antiseptic treatment of wounds; his successor Sir William Macewen had pioneered thoracic and brain surgery and Murdoch Cameron, Professor of Midwifery, demonstrated that caesarean section could save the lives of mothers and babies. It was a great tradition.

When the Glasgow vacancy occurred, it was suggested to Ian that he might consider applying and he agreed. Some months passed and nothing happened. Then one evening he received a mysterious summons to call at a certain house in Bryanston Square. There he found a rather vague, white-haired gentleman struggling into evening dress. This was Sir Hector Hetherington, Principal and Vice-Chancellor of the University of Glasgow and, at that time, Chairman of the Vice Chancellors of the United Kingdom.

Sir Hector asked Ian a few inconsequential questions and then apologised that he had to go for a very important dinner engagement. Again some months passed and the suspense was awful. Eventually it was resolved by another autocratic summons, this time in the form of an air ticket to Glasgow where he met with Sir Hector and various senior professors of the University in an informal interview over tea. On concluding this, Sir Hector said, "I believe you are interested in art. I would like you to come and see a picture we have recently acquired for the Glasgow Art Gallery. It will be closed by now, but don't worry, I'll have it opened". This exercise in academic power greatly impressed Ian. The Principal and professor-elect went down to the Art Gallery at Kelvingrove and the picture they saw was "Christ of St John of the Cross" by Salvador Dali, which was then a very controversial item. It had been bought by Dr Tom Honeyman, the Director of the Art Gallery, at the extravagant price of £8,200, which had caused an enormous public outcry.

Ian said goodbye and awaited events. He was very impressed by Sir Hector – and not without reason. Sir Hector was described by someone who knew him well as "a hard man with kid gloves" who, beneath that air of smiling, paternalistic benignity was one of the most ruthless and successful academic politicians of the twentieth century. Sir Hector treated the university as a personal fiefdom. He had no time for large committees and made all the vital decisions himself. He even controlled some of his professors' spare time. He had a humorous side and his favourite recreation was golf. His secretary kept a list of the golfing professors and, if Hector could see a minimum of two hours free, she telephoned them in turn until one was found who would "undertake an important duty for the university by getting the Principal into the fresh air and clearing his mind of all issues except the task in hand of getting the ball in the hole".

Hector Hetherington was appointed Principal of the University in 1936 and many hopes were placed on his capacity to revive "an institution in distress". He was admirably suited to the task. Born in Auchterarder in 1888, a Glasgow graduate in classics, economics and philosophy, he had held many academic and administrative posts and had been Vice-Chancellor of the University of Liverpool. He arrived in Glasgow in 1936 determined to make his mark on his alma mater. He led the University for twenty-five years.

From the start, Hetherington filled vacant senior positions by recruiting the most talented people he could find. Despite the difficulties caused by the war, he held on to this vision of the highest quality staff, particularly in science and medicine. One of his objectives was to place all clinical departments of the medical school in the charge of full-time professors, paid by the university at a rate high enough to make outside earnings unnecessary. As a result, academic medicine strode forward into the post-war years with increasing vigour and confidence. The University took the view that it was research and not didactic ability that gave the "vital inspiration so necessary to undergraduate and postgraduate education".

Glasgow had, in addition to the University, an independent tradition which stressed that it was clinical work that was central to medical education. Senior doctors remained sceptical of the reforms which they saw as a potentially fatal threat to traditional medical education and practice, founded on the rock of clinical experience. Eventually, understanding between the two points of view was reached. It was evolution not revolution. As the university approached its five hundredth birthday in 1951, Hetherington and the university staff had much of which to be proud. The only shadow was the theft of the "Stone of Destiny" from Westminster Abbey by a group of Nationalist students. This incurred Royal disapproval. But Glasgow students are always unpredictable.

The policy of talent spotting continued and in Ian Donald the Principal found someone whose qualities were ideally suited to

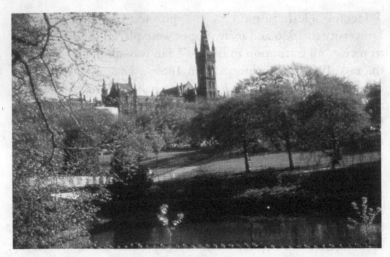

Glasgow University

his plan. He realised that a new teaching maternity hospital was essential to Glasgow. He promised this to Ian, who agreed with enthusiasm. All that Hetherington had to do then was to persuade (or rather instruct) the Secretary of State for Scotland to confirm the appointment. The Secretary of State was involved because this was a government appointment. To improve medical education the Crown had funded several new medical chairs in the early nineteenth century, including Midwifery (1815). These 'Regius Chairs' were not entirely popular at that time because the Government paid inadequate salaries and made no contribution to expenses. But things were different in the 1950s. The title of 'Regius Professor' was a grand one and Ian was very proud of his commission signed personally by the Queen. "In London", he used to say, "teaching hospitals keep their professor in a cupboard and bring him out only on occasion, to meet visitors. In America, the guy who plays the piano in a brothel is called "professor". But in Scotland, a Regius Professor is a king, and 'There's such divinity doth hedge a king, That treason can but peep to what it would'". It seemed that Sir Hector Hetherington was not alone in desiring control of all beneath him.

Glasgow Obstetrics
in the "Fifties"

The arrival of Professor Ian Donald in 1954 made an immediate impact on the Glasgow Royal Maternity Hospital.[1] Tall, impressive, with brilliant red hair and a rather leonine facial expression, he had a haughty aristocratic manner which was foreign to the inbred Glasgow scene. He looked rather like an English colonial administrator who had arrived to civilise the natives. This impression was emphasised by his occasional wearing of a monocle, although hauteur dissolved into laughter when it fell into his soup!

Those not in the intimacy of "C" unit, which he led, observed with cynical amusement how he sat in the centre of the long side of the table in the traditional hospital dining room with his juniors ranged to right and left. Those on his right hand looked left and those on his left looked right. It was a testimony to his personal magnetism that all of them seemed to hang on his every word. He had arrived to challenge the obstetric establishment and much of what he said was provoking.

He was, however, heir to a long tradition. The great clinical experience that had accumulated in Glasgow was the result of much social change. In the eighteenth century, Glasgow was a pleasant, prosperous academic town in rural surroundings, rather like Oxford, and was centred on its twelfth century cathedral and the elegant renaissance buildings of its university.

The nineteenth century brought change to Glasgow like a whirlwind. Demand for labour caused a dramatic rise in

---

1 Popularly referred to as "The Rottenrow". There was nothing rotten about the name, which dated from mediaeval times, being a translation of the Gaelic Rattad'n Righ or the French Route de Roi, the street the kings progressed along to the cathedral.

population. Great wealth was accumulated and great poverty endured. Coal, steam power and attendant inventions, such as the blast furnace, created heavy industry and the demand for labour caused a dramatic rise in population. The rapid explosion of population (fourteen-fold in less than a century) created Glasgow's greatest public health problem – lack of adequate housing. The centre of the city was described as "An accumulated mass of squalid wretchedness, where is concentrated everything which is dissolute, loathsome and pestilential". Never was there greater need for maternity services. The Glasgow Maternity Hospital opened in 1834.

For the next hundred years and more, the problems caused by contracted pelvis dominated Glasgow obstetrics, becoming latterly almost an obsession. This was not surprising, for rickets was rampant among the children of the poorer districts. Industrial pollution was everywhere: buildings became black with soot and frequently a pall of darkness descended on the city, cutting out the sunlight and preventing the synthesis of vitamin D. These atmospheric conditions combined with an inadequate diet and poor housing produced the women whose distorted pelves adorn obstetric museums, a grim reminder of an unlovely past.

The surgical solution to the problem was caesarean section, but this was a very dangerous operation with a death rate of seventy to eighty percent until the 1880s when Murdoch Cameron made it safe. Murdoch Cameron was Regius Professor of Midwifery from 1894 to 1927. His work opened a new era in obstetrics. The technique of classical caesarean section was further refined by his son Sam, who was assistant to his father and later Regius Professor of Midwifery from 1934 to 1943. The Camerons, father and son, were both practical men, direct and richly Scots in speech. Sam Cameron was an exceptionally rapid operator, but taught his juniors that simplicity of method and a sound knowledge of anatomy were more important than speed. He was also the author of an important and influential book, the *Glasgow Manual of Obstetrics*.

Another of Murdoch Cameron's assistants further developed the operation of caesarean section and achieved international fame. He was Dr JM Munro Kerr, eloquent and aristocratic in manner and a fluent and indefatigable medical author, whose *Operative Obstetrics* remains a classic. Unfortunately, Sam Cameron and Munro Kerr did not have a friendly relationship and their assistants formed rival camps. Petty medical feuds abounded. These divisions were eventually healed by Ian's predecessor, Professor Lennie.

Robert Aim Lennie (1889–1961) had a military background, having served in the RAMC with distinction in World War One and, in World War Two, as full Colonel RAMC, he commanded the Military Hospital at Drymen, near Loch Lomond. He was appointed Regius Professor of Midwifery in 1946. Not surprisingly, he had a military bearing as he delivered his lectures. He was a great obstetrical conservative and castigated many modern trends as "meddlesome midwifery". A quotation that sticks in the memory is, "The modern obstetrician is a membrane-puncturing episiotomising radio-caesareanist". Despite his Colonel Blimp type of conservation, Robert Lennie was personally kind and humorous and it was he who paved the way for Ian by creating a friendly hospital. He brought together the rival factions on the staff and visits to the Killermont golf course were very therapeutic. By 1954, all the three medical units in the hospital were talking to each other.

Dr John Hewitt, the head of "B" unit was a reserved and thoughtful man who devoted much research to pre-eclampsia in cooperation with Dr Harold Sheehan (of Sheehan's syndrome) and Dr ADT Govan, both obstetric pathologists of international renown. "A" unit was headed by the Muirhead Professor (with gynaecology at the Royal Infirmary). He was David Fyfe Anderson, who had a distinguished early career assisting Emil Novak at Johns Hopkins Hospital, Baltimore, USA. He was very much a "dour Scot" (although not without humour) and contributed little to medical literature, although his use (in the 1950s) of spinal anaesthesia (administered by himself) for caesarean section and magnesium sulphate for eclampsia have now become popular.

The Glasgow Royal Maternity Hospital had another great advantage: the outstanding ability of its midwives. A series of distinguished matrons and district sisters ensured the highest standards of practice. More than half of the deliveries took place outside hospital, often in slum surroundings, where the midwives and junior doctors always received a warm welcome. In 1954 the nursing care in the hospital was organised by a marvellous trio: Miss Renwick (Matron), Miss Raeside (Deputy) and Miss Burrows (Principal Tutor). The Medical Superintendent was Colonel Jebb (ex-Indian Medical Service), assisted by the Hospital Secretary, Mr Methven (a lawyer) and one or two typists. Medical administration had not yet become a growth industry.

Into this busy but traditional atmosphere erupted Ian Donald, a young, irreverent, red-haired professor from London who, like St Paul (one of his favourite authors) wanted to turn the world upside down.

Hector MacLennan was the senior member of "C" unit (he had been on the staff for twenty years) when Ian arrived and was undoubtedly a great help to him in those early days, making things easy for him and keeping him out of trouble. Handsome, impressive and histrionic, he could have been a great actor, a quality he shared with Ian Donald. He was widely read and was a splendid after-dinner speaker and raconteur. He was President of the RCOG in 1965 when the Congress of Obstetrics and Gynaecology took place in Glasgow and he carried out his duties with great style. He had a very fashionable and aristocratic private practice, although he was as courteous to a "wee Glesca' buddie" as to a duchess.

Hector loved his aristocratic contacts. On one occasion, he emerged from his house to go off shooting in a highland estate togged up in Inverness cape and shooting hat, and encountered his neighbour, the renowned Glasgow comic actor, Jimmy Logan. Jimmy remarked "Hey Hector, there's only the wan (one) coamic in this street!".

After his retirement, Sir Hector, as he then was, received many honours and chaired a number of important medical committees. His charm, diplomacy, powers of persuasion and acute mind were tremendous assets. Outside medicine, he was invited to be the first Chairman of the Scottish Tourist Board from 1969 to 1974. The honour that gave him greatest pleasure was his appointment as Lord High Commissioner to the General Assembly of the Church of Scotland for 1975 and 1976. As the Queen's representative, he was accorded Royal honours, so that as he was driven along Princes Street all the traffic lights turned to green and when he appeared on the balcony of Holyrood Palace the band played "God Save the Queen". No one could have played this part better. Hector was generous, approachable and enjoyed life to the full. He always noted the best qualities in people and was ever ready to help a colleague. He had an agile mind and an extraordinary memory for detail. His native caution, added to his wisdom and judgement, made him the ideal person from whom to seek an opinion and, above all, he was kindly. Ian Donald was indeed lucky to have such a wise advisor.

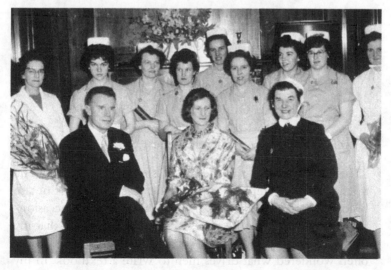

Prizegiving GRMH
Ian, Alix and Miss Renwick (Matron)

"Sharing Enthusiasm"

A textbook – and a teacher – with a difference

While in Hammersmith, Ian Donald had been working on a textbook of obstetrics, which he finished in September 1954, just after his appointment to the Glasgow Chair. It was quite unlike anything that had appeared before and exploded on the academic scene like a display of fireworks. We who were young read it from cover to cover like a novel. We could not put it down. We shall now let Ian speak for himself and our readers may begin to know how we felt as we read *Practical Obstetric Problems*.

The book begins with a dedication:

"To all who have known doubt, perplexity and fear as
I have known them,
To all who have made mistakes as I have,
To all whose humility increases with their knowledge
of this most fascinating subject

THIS BOOK IS DEDICATED".

The preface follows in equally dramatic style.

"The art of teaching is the art of sharing enthusiasm. The teacher must, therefore, love what he teaches if he is not to become "as a tingling cymbal". If, then, exuberance occasionally bubbles through the pages of this book, I know that my past students will understand, and I ask no forgiveness. I have often wondered what drives men to write a textbook. In my case it was the persuasiveness of my publisher."

— 20 —

He felt, and of course he is right, that there was a place for a book of a practical sort, which would appeal to the clinician who lives in the rough and tumble of it all, as well as to aspirants for additional diplomas in the subject.

> We agreed upon a strategic size, and therefore, we hope, upon a palatable price, but apart from that I was given a completely free hand. I gladly accepted the excuse to omit the inevitable dreary irrelevance of such matters as ovulation, menstruation, conception, infertility, diagnosis of pregnancy and the early development of the ovum, which can be found in most textbooks of midwifery making them heavy upon the knee as well as upon the mental digestion of the reader. Having got rid of this burden I found myself free to get down to the real business of midwifery. In doing so I may or may not have pleased my public (if any) but I certainly pleased myself. The would-be pianist does not struggle through his Beethoven because of the imagined needs of a hypothetical audience. His efforts are owed to the Master. It is in this spirit that I have written and I can only hope that some will find it infectious.

It certainly was infectious, and became world famous. After due acknowledgement to colleagues who had helped him, Ian concluded his preface as follows:

> It would not be fair, in all these acknowledgements, to omit mention of my long-suffering wife and family, who have put up with me and my book for so many months. Most of the time that I gave to the task was really their time and their contribution has been the calm with which they have managed to surround my domestic life and without which I would surely have failed. In retrospect it has been worthwhile and if, in the pages that follow, I have at times provoked, instructed and amused, then I am content.

Ian's high-minded ideals about teaching did not necessarily appeal to all his Glasgow colleagues. His fellow professor, David Fyfe Anderson, on casually meeting him in a hospital corridor, remarked in his usual dry and possibly humorous way, "Oh, Ian, I would like a read of your book". This conveyed to an observer that DFA had not read it and certainly had no intention of buying it!

But lots of people bought it and were entranced by its unique flavour and by the character of a medical author who could write, "Dullness is as much out of place in a textbook as anywhere else, for not only should books be informative they should be read with enjoyment. Textbooks have been referred to as 'storehouses of unexpurgated tradition'. Understatement is often referred to as 'masterly' while overstatement is usually dismissed as poetic licence, if not worse. But poetry lingers in the mind".

Had diagnostic ultrasound never been developed, Ian Donald would be remembered as a great clinical teacher. *Practical Obstetric Problems* had an enormous impact internationally and, through it, the name of Donald became as famous on the banks of the Nile and the Ganges as on those of the Clyde. The book acquired the status of Holy Writ and it was a particular irritation when one was teaching foreign postgraduates in their home countries and wanted to express a personal point of view on something important.

The crushing reply from them would be "But Ian Donald he say on page 342 –". There was no answer.

Practical Obstetric Problems went into five editions, the last of which appeared in 1979. With advancing knowledge in many spheres it inevitably gained weight, but succeeded in remaining personal in tone. When Ian wrote the preface to the first edition he wondered what it was that drove a man to write a textbook. A friend supplied the cynical answer that it was in the hope of learning something about the subject. Ian commented, "I know that he was right. There has been much to learn since the last edition and, in order to keep the book within manageable size, every possible scrap of dead wood has had to be cut away". But this last edition went to 1071 pages, with masses of excellent illustrations and long lists of references after each chapter, in which the name "DONALD, I", needless to say, appeared frequently. He was never a man to hide his light under a bushel and over the years the young maverick professor of the 1950s had become a great international figure and a "grand old man"– but one with a difference. He had lost none of his incisiveness: he retained his streaks of mischief and the tireless self-publicity, which kept him going.

The drama of obstetric emergencies is well conveyed and clear directions for action are given. The text is enlivened with clinical anecdotes, in some of which Ian frankly admits his mistakes. All this contrasts with modern medical publications that seek political or statistical correctness in preference to clarity and direct contact with the reader. Most of the encyclo-paedic material presented about antenatal complications, medical disorders in pregnancy and the management of labour and delivery is still relevant today, particularly in developing countries but, of course, the last quarter century has brought many changes, such as the decline of some medical compli-cations and the increased safety of caesarean section, which has made much manipulative obstetrics unnecessary.

We believe that the personality of Ian Donald is best delivered in his own words, in which he was never lacking and we enclose the following quotations from his book.

The Scope of Antenatal Care

As the hazards to the mother of pregnancy and labour continue to recede, so too have those to the fetus come to be recognised more acutely during its intra-uterine existence. The first 38 weeks of human life spent in the allegedly protected environment of the amniotic sac are medically more eventful and more fraught with danger and accident than the next 38 years of the lifespan of most human individuals. The scope therefore of antenatal care is widening rapidly in this direction.

We are only on the threshold of a new and far more important type of antenatal care than hitherto and, inasmuch as prevention is always better than cure, it is the function of antenatal care to reduce the need for desperate measures at the time of delivery. Unfortunately the present situation leaves little room for more than "divine discontent", since we cannot yet match the recent improvement in labour room tactics with those of antenatal care itself. Nevertheless, gone are the days, I hope, of the hospital "cram clinic" which treated its patients like machine parts on an assembly line, being mainly concerned with the prevention of eclampsia, the correction of normal presentation and recognising disproportion, if it could.

The ability to see 60 patients in 65 minutes is a type of pre-war insult – according to the patient little more recognition than the status of an appendage of her gravid uterus and its contents. To a woman who may have waited an hour or more in an unattractive waiting space in even less attractive company, the rapid exposure of her bulging abdominal surface and the overhearing of a few muttered remarks to some assistant writing notes, followed by a hurried dismissal, must have seemed a travesty of medical care as indeed it was. Yet such tactics have not entirely died out.

Domiciliary Delivery

Whatever the merits of this, and they are considerable, there is no doubt that domiciliary midwifery is dying in the more highly developed populations of the world socially, such as the white population of the United States, Sweden and Australia, much in the same way as traditional tonsillectomy on the kitchen table is more or less gone for good. It is also the avowed policy in Great Britain to provide maternity beds for every pregnant woman in the land, if she so wishes, and most do. This trend would have more to be said for it if many hospitals were not rather grisly, out-of-date places with out-of-date thinking, especially on matters like visiting and patient freedom, and occasionally run by a human species of dragon, and if only food in all hospitals could be treated with the dignity and intelligent artistry which cooking deserves and if private nursing homes were not often so ruinously expensive. Discipline in hospital which varies from the irksome to the terrifying can almost be reminiscent of one's days at boarding school in childhood. It is essential in all new hospital planning that these objections be vigorously and consciously overcome as they have been in our new Queen Mother's Hospital, where open visiting is allowed and where children are allowed to visit their mothers and "see the new baby".

Irregular dismissals, against medical advice, are therefore rare indeed and we keep no such register; nor is any notice, other than a direction notice, allowed to be displayed for the instruction of patients, including futile restrictions on smoking; the latter only encourages secret smoking in lavatories and bathrooms to the detriment of the drains and the general hygiene of the place.

Abortion Legislation

The abortion scene has altered drastically in both the United Kingdom and the United States since virtually an abortion on demand principle, at least for those who can pay for it, has been legalised in both countries. This may not have been the intention of most of our legislators but is nevertheless a matter of fact.

An attempt to provide safeguards against wanton and indiscriminate abortion was made in the British Abortion Act of 1967 but these were doomed to failure because of the breadth of interpretation which could be applied to the working of the Act. In the briefest possible terms British law does not now regard it as unlawful to abort a woman if two practitioners of more that a few years standing "in good faith" consider such is necessary for the following reasons:

in the interests of the woman's life;

1. in the interests of her health, mental as well as physical;
2. in the interests of the health, mental and physical, of other existing children, and
3. if there is a risk of serious fetal handicap.

The operative phrase here is "in good faith". This is at sometimes less evident than at others.

One good point was the control of premises where legalised abortions could be carried out and another was the insistence of notification.

In so far as this last condition is fulfilled some useful statistical information might emerge as in other countries. In the United Kingdom the annual legalised abortion rate continued to rise steadily every year reaching approximately 156,000 for England and Wales in 1973, although about one-third of these were private patients from abroad – a form of invisible export which does the British medical profession little credit. It is difficult to see at what point this rising curve will level out but my guess, to judge from other countries with similar cultural standards, would be at about one-third of the rate for all births. In other words, a quarter of a million annually. This sort of thing is not medicine; it is sociological scavenging and will not be discussed further in this book, nor will its social implications. Volumes of ink and rhetoric have been spilt already.

Our own personal hostility to abortion on so-called "social grounds" as a method of long-stop contraception is modified when confronted with scientific evidence of serious disability which may threaten the intra-uterine baby's chance of a fulfilled life, particularly mental and spiritual fulfilment in so far as these can be foreseen. This raises an ethical issue on which the opinions of doctors can never be uniformly agreed. In the face of such incontrovertible evidence as a rising rubella antibody titre or a cast-iron genetic diagnosis of major disability reached by amniocentesis, I think the patient has a right to know the facts and to make some personal choice in the matter. This is altogether different from abortion on demand, whatever politicians or governments in their ill-informed ignorance may attempt to dictate.

Management of Labour

O, that a man might know
The end of this day's business ere it come!
But it sufficeth that the day will end,
And then the end is known.

SHAKESPEARE, *Julius Caesar*, Act V, Sc.1

A labour which is unduly prolonged is likely to give rise to one or more of three types of distress, namely maternal, fetal, or "obstetricians' distress". Of the three the last may be easily the most dangerous! These cases tax clinical judgement, often to the limit, and then a second opinion, come freshly on the scene, is worth a lot. In hospital practice this is usually automatic, but in domiciliary work importuning relatives may easily distract judgement already wavering in the cause of plain humanity, with the result that intervention is often prematurely, ill-advisedly or unnecessarily undertaken.

Dawn should not rise twice upon the same labour. Nowadays we would regard any labour lasting more than 24 hours as pathological and, in the case of the multiparous patient, positively sinister. All such cases need the facilities of a properly staffed and equipped obstetrical unit.

We have come a long way since the days in the 1930s when my first obstetrical case laboured for five days (and I too!) and although she delivered herself spontaneously in the end, she became acutely psychotic a few days later and was removed to a mental institution where, so I learned, she did not do well. These were days when we were more concerned with maternal survival than fetal wellbeing. Caesarean section, usually classical, carried a mortality of not less than 5 per cent and the philosophy of those days was that the first baby at least was always expendable in the interests of the mother's obstetrical future. I first came into obstetrics towards the end of a truly horrific period of maternal hazard and suffering and my memory is more deeply engraved with the disasters of those days than it is with any subsequent successes.

The Vacuum Extractor (Ventouse)

Ian Donald was keen to try anything new. The idea of vacuum extraction of the baby was not new but was revived by Professor Tage Malmström of Gothenburg in the 1950s. It became popular in Europe while conventional forceps delivery was still universal in Britain. Ian Donald visited Professor Smoeck's department in Brussels in 1961 and observed that the vacuum extractor had completely replaced the obstetric forceps since 1958, without any increase in the caesarean section rate. Also in 1961, at the World Congress of Gynaecology and Obstetrics in Vienna, thirty-five papers were produced describing experience with Malmström's extractor. Ian was determined to try it. Unfortunately, Fothergill and Chalmers of Worcester pipped us to the post with a publication in *The Practitioner*, also in 1961, but Ian Donald, with JW in the labour ward, pressed on amid ribald remarks about "suck it and see!". The great benefit of the technique was that most cases were delivered under local anaesthesia.

Such was Ian's curiosity that, as was his wont, he tried out the vacuum extractor on himself, placing it on his brow and leaving the typical "chignon" characteristic of the instrument. He had to explain the resultant bruising in the days ahead, to his embarrassment. Another bizarre experiment was described by Ian in his textbook.

I have deliberately sought to measure the traction forces which can be applied before the cup pulls away from the scalp. For this purpose I waited, and had to wait a long time, for a fresh stillbirth which occurred in a case of hydrops late one Saturday afternoon. I hurriedly made in my workshop a sort of miniature lavatory seat to fit the baby's head exactly, wedged the head into this "brim" and applied the ventouse in the standard manner.

I then rigged the whole thing up in the mortuary so that weights could be applied directly to the ventouse in increasing amounts and at 23 lb (10 kg) the vacuum broke and the cup came off. This is a very much smaller force than is usually applied with forceps as has been described earlier and constitutes one of the great safety factors in this operation.

In clinical use Ian commented:

The direction of pull is largely determined by what looks most rewarding and since adopting this principle the success rate has improved enormously. To deliver a woman within half an hour, after many days of tedious and unrewarding labour, is a very satisfying experience and much to be preferred to caesarean section or forceps. Willocks (1962) who, in my department, has used the apparatus more extensively than any of us, has listed the following major indications:

1. To deliver some cases of fetal distress occurring late in the first stage of labour;
2. To complete delivery in some cases of uterine inertia late in the first stage;
3. As an alternative to trial of forceps in some multiparae in whom second-stage delay is associated with deflexion

and malposition of the fetal head at the pelvic brim or high in the pelvic cavity, and

4. To rotate and deliver the head in many cases of occipito-transverse and posterior positions.

He also adds that the ventouse may be used instead of forceps in the second stage and I agree that it makes a very pleasant alternative to the simple low forceps operation.

I had the gratifying experience of delivering one of my own staff midwives with the ventouse after an hour-and-a-half of profitless second staging and her comment after delivery was, "I am so glad I managed it all myself". She did not even know at the time that she had been delivered by ventouse. I wonder if one could say that same even for the easiest of low forceps operations and I felt this was tribute indeed to the gentleness of the method.

Postpartum Haemorrhage

"If you can fill the unforgiving minute with sixty seconds worth of distance run"

KIPLING

This is indeed the unforgiving stage of labour, and in it there lurks more unheralded treachery than in both the other stages of labour combined. The normal case can, within a minute, become abnormal and successful delivery can turn swiftly to disaster. The obstetrician's judgement must be sure and swift, and errors of commission carry with them penalties as great, or greater, than those of omission. Increasing experience serves only to sharpen one's alertness during this stage, and there is no room for complacency in any case, however normal, until the placenta has been delivered for at least half an hour, with the uterus well retracted and with minimal bleeding.

> It is far more important to understand the physiology of this stage of labour than to know the mechanisms of the second stage and the only safe management is one based upon this knowledge.

These few excerpts give an idea of the flavour of the book. "Too personal" for some but for those with imagination, it is still worth a read. Ian Donald did believe sincerely that "the art of teaching is the art of sharing enthusiasm".

The Western Infirmary
Wards G9 and 10

The Professorial Department of Gynaecology was in the Western Infirmary, adjacent to the University on Gilmorehill. The proposal to build a new hospital in the West of Glasgow originated in 1845, when the University Court was impelled to contemplate a move westwards because the College buildings in High Street were inadequate to meet the demands resulting from the city's unprecedented growth, and the surroundings of the university had deteriorated. Construction of the new building at Gilmorehill, described as a "charming green rising ground far to the west", began in 1867 and it was ready for occupation (although not yet complete) in 1870, when the professors were photographed on the Lion and Unicorn Stair of the Old College, a dinner was held in the Fore Hall, the loving cup was passed round with the appropriate sentiment and "Resurgat in gloria Alma Mater" and "Auld Lang Syne" were sung. Next day, the historic Old College was handed over to the railway company.

The Royal Infirmary had provided admirable convenient facilities for clinical teaching but was regarded as too remote from the new university site, and adjacent ground was purchased to accommodate a new hospital. It became apparent that, apart from university requirements, the hospital needed to act as a second general infirmary for the city and, as the public was contributing generously for this purpose, their needs were also important.

The Western Infirmary opened in November 1874 when there were 110 inpatients and over the next three years their number was to average 153. A department of diseases of women was opened in 1877. The infirmary expanded greatly in the twentieth century but provision for gynaecology remained sparse. The department had only one ward of twenty beds, although it had one of the best operating theatres in the hospital. Good service was given but the waiting list reached distressing magnitude.

Things changed in 1954 when Ian Donald was appointed Regius Professor. For gynaecology, the Western gave him its pleasantest wards, forty-eight beds on the top floor of the New Wing. Full use was made of them during Ian's reign. The only anxiety the administration had was our undue use of extra beds, which we needed to demolish the massive waiting list. The history of the Western Infirmary 1874–1974 records that Donald "built a fine team whose members have each done more than their excellent clinical work". Wallace Barr has a creditable textbook to his name; John MacVicar, distinguished for his contribution to the development of his subject in the new Nairobi School, has resigned this year on appointment to the foundation Chair of Obstetrics and Gynaecology in the University of Leicester; James Willocks has been described as a "great loss to the Church but this is a tribute to his capacity for scholastic exposition and in no way detracts from his medical distinction".

The gynaecological department of the Western Infirmary was situated in the third and top floor of the 'University' block. It consisted of two large wards, G9 and 10, housing together forty-eight patients.

On the ground floor were the wards of Professor Edward J Wayne. These were linked to the Gardner Institute of Medicine, a research department which at that time was devoting much effort to the study and treatment of high blood pressure.

The middle floor was occupied by the Department of Surgery under the guidance of Sir Charles Illingworth, whose team was pre-eminent in the management of gastrointestinal complaints and in whose department had been constructed a hyperbaric oxygen pressure chamber for the treatment of respiratory problems and for the repressurising of deep-sea divers at risk from 'the bends'.

Wards G9 and 10 were of the old-fashioned "Nightingale" type, each being a huge single room with a large long table in the centre. The patients lay along either side of the ward and privacy, when required, was provided by mobile screens which were dragged round the bed by the nursing or medical staff. These were later replaced by curtains on a fixed rail about each bed. Toilet and bathing facilities were provided at the far end of the ward, where there was also a balcony in which ambulant patients could sit and enjoy the fresh air. To our knowledge it was seldom used for this purpose, but frequently for smoking. There was also one single room kept for a patient who may be seriously ill or dying or was perhaps a medical or nursing colleague.

Each ward was presided over by the sister, whose office lay at the proximal end of the ward. The senior sister at the time of Ian's arrival was a gracious lady of the old school. Helen Batchelor found the new professor somewhat strange, but they soon established a *modus vivendi*. The sister's office was the nerve centre of the ward where sister or her deputy could be relied upon to provide up-to-the-minute information about each patient and where problem cases were discussed, usually followed by the provision of morning coffee.

Each ward also had a ward maid who was responsible for the cleanliness and tidiness of the ward. She was usually a typical "wee Glasgow wumman" who took a fierce pride in her work and made a much better job of it than the faceless ever-changing contract cleaners who are nowadays responsible. She ran errands for the patients and carried out all sorts of little tasks, besides being the purveyor of scurrilous gossip mostly about the medical staff.

A ward round was carried out each day by a consultant attended by his registrar and the house surgeon, together with those medical students who were not in theatre or in the out-patient department. Each consultant was responsible for his own patients, whom he would have seen initially in the outpatient clinic and referred from there to his own operating list. On the ward round, however, he saw all patients in the ward and dealt with any problem causing concern to the sister or house surgeon.

One part of the organisation remains to be described: the Office, which was really the nerve centre of the unit. It had three occupants, the admissions' clerk and two secretaries who worked tirelessly to maintain a steady, up-to-date stream of dismissal letters to be sent to each patient's family doctor at the time of her discharge from hospital. These women were also responsible for obtaining laboratory reports and filing them into the case records. They had to maintain a close liaison with the outpatient department and the hospital records office and were also required to chase up the consultant staff in order to 'persuade' them to dictate letters promptly so that they could be typed and despatched without delay. It is no exaggeration to say that the efficiency of the unit depended upon the dedication of these women to the job in hand.

Every Saturday there was the GRAND WARD ROUND. This was an institution established by the Professor soon after his arrival in Glasgow. It really was a remarkable occasion, in that all members of the unit from the most senior to the most junior convened voluntarily each week out of normal working hours to consider all the patients under their care. The procession, headed by the Professor, stopped at each patient's bed and the details of her case were presented by the house surgeon, with or without the benefit of case notes. Many of the cases required only cursory attention and a word of greeting to the patient from Ian Donald, but 'problem' or interesting cases brought the procession to a halt to be followed by a detailed discussion. The ward round thus made for clinical efficiency and provided a forum for debate, each case providing an intellectual challenge in which diagnostic priority and merits of potential treatments were discussed with some fervour. There were splendid theatrical moments and the whole thing was strangely reminiscent of a scene from Richard Gordon's "Doctor in the House", in the film of which Sir Lancelot Spratt, played by James Robertson Justice, conducts a ward round along similar lines.

To quote from Gordon's book of the same name published in 1952. "The round was held every Thursday morning at ten o'clock and had the same effect on the ward as an admiral's inspection of a small warship. Preparations for the visit began about five in the morning. The night nurses started the long business of sprucing up the ward and when her day staff arrived at seven, the energy given to preparing the long room was increased ten-fold, so that nothing offensive should fall on the great man's eye. At nine, the senior house surgeon in a fresh white jacket looked in for a worried whispered conversation with sister to be certain that everything had been done. The ward, by ten, was silent, orderly and odourless."

In the Western Infirmary similar preparations were made, but the grand ward round did not finish with the exit of medical staff from the ward. Discussion continued even after the round. Dr Alistair Miller recalls, "It was a Saturday morning after the ward round and the next week's admissions were being looked at and the lists planned. (How different from now!) Ian Donald was in expansive form and there was quite a crowd, as usual. I recollect a lot of laughter from those days, which grew out of the regular get-togethers of the whole unit, in the hospital or in adjacent hostelries, 'The Rubaiyat', the 'Skandia' and later the 'Stirling Castle'.

Life with Ian Donald was never dull and he enjoyed these social occasions, which built up the sense of teamwork nowadays lost by modern bureaucratic management.

The "Nightingale" wards have now disappeared from most hospitals, to be replaced by small three- or four-bedded wards and single rooms. We think this is a cause for regret, as the sense of community and exchange of views across the ward boosted morale and contributed much to the recovery of the patient.

Another factor, which, of course, does not apply nowadays, was that patients spent a much longer time in hospital post-operatively. Minor surgical cases went home on the day after operation but "majors" were detained for seven or eight days or longer if they had a problem such as a wound being slow to heal or a bladder difficult to empty. Such cases nowadays are sent home before the complications arise and become the responsibility of the GP or home-visiting nurses. Inevitably, a number of them have to be readmitted for the care they should have been given before leaving hospital. This is just one of the several 'advances' in treatment introduced with the advent of the 'NHS modernisation' but, in the opinion of many older doctors, it simply shifts the responsibility for patient care on to other shoulders outwith the hospital and 'massages' the figures for hospital admission.

The Cutting Edge

In the operating theatre

Prior to the Second World War, gynaecological surgery fell within the province of the general surgeon, who confined himself to the removal of large pelvic tumours, with or without the uterus, and to the repair of damage caused by prolonged labours or traumatic deliveries. However, during the immediate post-war years, gynaecology emerged as a separate subject and was linked with midwifery, to be recognised as obstetrics and gynaecology.

This change was facilitated by the establishment in London of the Royal College of Obstetricians and Gynaecologists, which laid down rules for the training, examination and graduation of those doctors who specialised in this subject. In medical schools it was then taught as a separate part of the curriculum to be undertaken in the later stages of the course and incorporated in the Final Examination with medicine and surgery.

In these early years, London was the principal teaching centre where the leading exponents of the subject worked in famous teaching hospitals and names like Victor Bonney, Comyns Berkeley and "Joe"Wrigley were attracting attention from all over the world. Bonney, in particular, was notable for his book which described the full range of gynaecological operative procedures, beautifully illustrated with pencil drawings by his own hand.

When Donald came to the Chair in Glasgow in 1954, he was fortunate to have been trained and to have worked with these famous men.

Learning to be a surgeon is a slow process. The necessary knowledge can be obtained from books but mastering the technique requires 'hands on' practice and this is first obtained by assisting at operations carried out by a senior colleague until one becomes proficient enough to be allowed to operate under supervision. In the Western Infirmary, the final 'passing out' procedure was to have the Professor act as assistant. As can be imagined, this was a most intimidating experience for the embryo surgeon although, for the most part, Ian Donald was patient and kindly. He was not the best assistant, however, since he often became involved in conversation with the anaesthetist or other bystander. James Willocks recounts the story of his own baptism of fire when Ian Donald said mellifluously, "Now, Willocks, I want you to operate on the next case and I shall assist you as I would like to know if there is anything I should adopt into my own practice". On conclusion he declared fortissimo, "There is nothing in your technique that I would wish to adopt".

A similar experience was recorded by our long-time friend and colleague, Dr Alistair Miller. He writes, "I was a resident in the Western Infirmary, 1962–63. A case of ectopic pregnancy was admitted; they were not common then and the operation was often given to the current resident so that it could be included in his Membership book.

Ian Donald offered to take me through– 'shall I bellyache, Alistair or shall I just suffer in silence?'. I thought it would be better for me if he bellyached and the case went reasonably well. On about the fourth or fifth day, however, the wound burst, discharging a haematoma. I went to the Professor's room, shamefaced, to confess and received no sympathetic commiseration! 'Have you counted the clips?', he barked. I hadn't and did not know how many I had inserted in the first place. He insisted that the patient be sent to X-ray to ensure there were no clips left within the wound. Another lesson learned!"

The operating theatre in the Western Infirmary was separated from the wards by a corridor about fifty metres in length. It was an old-fashioned spacious room with a huge skylight window extending along all of one side and an upstairs gallery for the better viewing of the operation by students and visitors. On one side were the staff changing rooms and on the other a room containing a large autoclave for sterilising the paraphernalia required for modern surgery. It was run by Sister Helen Abernethy: young, vivacious, humorous and "unflappable". Patients were anaesthetised in an anteroom before being taken into theatre.

Each of the four consultants (the Professor and Drs Barr, McVicar and Willocks) had an operating list who were patients taken from their own outpatient clinics so that they were familiar with the details of the case before surgery. Each consultant had his own registrar who assisted at the operation with the house surgeon.

The Professor's list was on a Thursday and often contained the most difficult and unusual cases. In these days the GPs who referred cases to the hospital regarded the Professor as the top clinical opinion and sent the most complicated and difficult cases for his outpatient opinion and thence to his theatre list (nowadays this does not necessarily apply as professors are often appointed on the strength of their research or laboratory credentials, so that they have no claim to wide experience or special skill in dealing with clinical, diagnostic or operative problems).

The Thursday list was seldom without incident. Anaesthetics were administered by not one but two of the hospitals most senior consultants, usually Dr James Crawford and Dr Hugh Wishart, who combined to produce the highest possible level of anaesthetic skill and postoperative recovery management. They regarded themselves as part of the gynaecological unit and, as they also possessed an acerbic wit and a shrewd capacity for assessing the surgical skills of the various operators, their comments and opinions added much to the interest and excitement of the proceedings.

It fell to me, WB, to be the principal assistant and for this there were two reasons. Firstly I was the most experienced. The second good reason for being there was that I could recognise the approach of the "Jesus Christ factor". Ian was not given to profanity and this was his only expletive under stress.

Ian Donald was a fine surgeon and it is a tribute to his skill and dedication that he insisted on undertaking the most difficult and complicated cases on Thursday mornings. However, as time progressed and his cardiac condition deteriorated, he sometimes found the physical strain well nigh intolerable. At moments of frustration, perhaps associated with a prolonged and difficult dissection, he would often express his exasperation with an explosive and long drawn out "Je-e-e-sus Christ"– a warning to all in the vicinity to take good care, that his displeasure was increasing, and that they should do nothing to aggravate his already shortening temper.

One such incident comes to mind. It concerned the Reverdin needle. This instrument was unknown to us in the North, but the Professor had been trained in its use in London and insistent on using it for all his abdominal cases. It consisted of a large handle attached to a needle, the eye of which could be opened and shut by a little device in the handle. When the needle had been put through the tissues, the eye was opened and it was the job of the assistant to thread the catgut or other suture material into the eye of the needle, which was then closed and the instrument extricated, bringing with it the suture. It sounds a simple enough procedure but in practice it caused problems. If the assistant was not practised in its use he was at great risk of incurring a severe laceration of his finger or at least a tear in his rubber glove, necessitating a delay until a substitute glove had been obtained and donned. This caused the inevitable "Je-e-e-sus Christ" as the Professor became more and more irascible. It also caused much secret hilarity on the part of Messrs Crawford and Wishart, who much enjoyed these Thursday morning adventures.

One particular incident comes to mind. On that occasion, a junior registrar had been promoted to principal assistant – a terrifying experience for one so young. He was wearing one of those disposable facemasks with an elastic loop over each ear. In his attempt to thread the Reverdin needle, his nose was almost buried in the wound and when the needle was extracted it caught the elastic of his mask. There was a moment of extreme crisis. The

Professor didn't realise what had caught the needle and as he pulled it to and fro he dragged the unfortunate registrar's head one way and the other until the elastic finally snapped. There was a mighty explosion of "Je-e-e-sus Christ" and nobody knew what would happen next. And then we laughed. We couldn't help it as the ridiculously farcical aspect of the situation struck us and, to his eternal credit, the Professor saw the funny side and joined in the hilarity. That young registrar is now himself a distinguished professor in a London teaching hospital and a world authority on obstetric ultrasound, but I am sure he has not forgotten the time he assisted Ian Donald.

A similar dramatic experience was recorded by Alistair Miller: "I was assisting Ian Donald in theatre (with Wallace Barr there, fortunately!) at a vaginal hysterectomy where, I thought, he was a little tense. This was a very easy case, however, and the tiny uterus fell out without difficulty. Having ligated the pedicles containing blood vessels; he had placed his usual additional ligatures on them to incorporate them into the vault of the vagina. By now he was talking volubly and he inadvertently cut one of the pedicles on my side of the table. When he noticed, he accused me, "You've cut my pedicle, Alistair!". "No", I protested, "you did". He replied, "Why would I do that?". It required WB's intervention to convince him that the long scissors he was using had done the damage. He continued to smoulder until the operation was safely concluded. These storms always passed very quickly and normal relations resumed. In general he was very good at listening to juniors".

The theatre had a gallery for students, also distinguished visitors. One memorable day we were visited by Sir Hector MacLennan, who sat in the gallery observing a complex operation. Something went wrong, the "Je-e-e-sus Christ!" factor came into play, but thanks to the calm assistance of WB all was put right. At this point Sir Hector observed suavely from the gallery, "Ian, I'll tell you how to avoid that mistake". The Professor, always the eternal student himself, asked mildly, "What is that, Hector?". Sir Hector replied "Take more care!". The proceedings dissolved in laughter. There was a great sense of 'cameraderie' in our department and it was often put to the test in theatre where we all helped each other.

The drama of theatre absorbed Ian completely. Another instance concerned JW who, in a more senior position, was first assistant in the first case on the list. He had got up in the morning feeling unwell and as the operation progressed, he had increasing and eventually unbearable pain. He said to the chief "I've got to go now. I'm not well". The chief remarked to his second assistant, the house surgeon, "Oh, Margaret, come round to the other side of the table and assist me". Meanwhile, JW was carted off to the ward side room (the first male patient in the gynaecology ward), had the indignity of having a stomach tube passed by the staff nurse and was rushed off to a surgical unit for an emergency operation for strangulated hernia. The professor remained oblivious, illustrating his single-mindedness for the job in hand.

As time went by and his health worsened, Ian Donald contributed personally to the drama of theatre even more. Assistants were on the alert for his dramatic departures from theatre, when we would find him lying flat out on one of the benches in the changing room. Those who did not know him well were surprised when he got up and continued a sprightly conversation.

On another occasion, during one of his breathless episodes, he created a minor sensation by marching into theatre like a deep-sea diver, with a large cylinder strapped to his back, supplying oxygen through a nasal catheter.

Ian Donald's inventive mind was seldom at rest. He was quick to seize on any new idea and when he heard of the laparoscope and 'keyhole surgery' he decided that he must see the instrument in action. Its main protagonist was Patrick Steptoe, who practised in Oldham and he and WB went there for a demonstration. As often happens on these occasions, the operation was a disastrous failure, but Donald was quick to appreciate its potential and arranged for a laparoscope to be purchased. Thereafter, many Thursday morning sessions were devoted to mastering the technique.

One of the difficulties was that the assistant had to hold the instrument steady while the Professor carried out the operation through a separate small incision. To dispense with the help of the assistant, he invented 'the snake', a flexible, multi-jointed tube which could be clamped to the operating table. It was not really a success, being heavy and clumsy and liable to collapse at critical moments, but it was another demonstration of the inventiveness of his mind.

Another illustration of his active, restless, enquiring mind was demonstrated when he devised his own method of *in vitro* fertilisation.

This involved the removal of an embryo from the fallopian tube in a case of ectopic pregnancy and transferring the intact ovum into the uterus of the infertile patient. This procedure required a masterpiece of synchronisation in theatre and the most careful preparation and timing.

Tragedy of tragedies! When the transfer of the ovum was taking place it slipped from his grasp and fell into his boot. The whole thing was a shambles and, in retrospect, was doomed to failure from the start, but it did not discourage the Professor from putting it to the test.

Television today, with its plethora of medical soap operas, has given many people the impression that operating theatres are daily the scene of high drama with frequent episodes of cardiac arrest or torrential haemorrhage requiring massive blood transfusion. While this may be the case in the casualty department of some hospitals, the average operating theatre in this country is less exciting. Much of the surgery and routine is repetitive and only rarely are there scenes of high drama. However, one such occasion does come to mind when the first and probably the only caesarean section was carried out in the Western Infirmary. We had been approached by the neurosurgeons, who had a patient with a leaking cerebral aneurysm. She was far advanced in pregnancy and they were afraid that the strain of labour would cause the aneurysm to rupture and they wanted her to have an elective section carried out in our theatre followed immediately by the brain surgery. Fortunately all went smoothly and rapidly. As soon as her abdomen was closed, her skull was opened and the leaking blood vessel tied off, so that the final outcome for mother and child was a happy one.

The Western Infirmary, as we knew it, is now long closed. We visited it recently and many memorable times were recalled. One of the most notable events was 'The Blitz' of 1960, which exemplified the team spirit existing in those days and so absent now. It occurred when it was reported to the Professor that the waiting list for minor operations numbered more than six hundred and that these patients were having to wait at least six months. "We'll have a Blitz then on the waiting list", he said and immediately set about organising it.

It was planned with military efficiency. Having secured the cooperation of the matron, to provide the additional nursing staff, and of the anaesthetic department, it was arranged that 200 minor operations would be carried out over a period of two weeks. Medical students were pressed into service as porters transporting the patients to and from the theatre where two surgeons, paired with two anaesthetists, worked in tandem to complete twenty minor operations per day.

There were no administrators to hamper the proceedings by quoting regulations regarding the statutory number of operations to be carried out per day and no trade union officials to protest at this 'misuse of labour' and the whole thing was an unqualified success. All concerned enjoyed a great sense of achievement, the waiting list was decimated and, above all, there was nobody to say it couldn't be done. The whole idea was conceived and inspired by the Professor and was typical of the man. Alas, it couldn't happen nowadays and perhaps this is why our National Health Service is limping along, overburdened with managers and administrators whose numbers have flourished alarmingly and who contribute nothing to the actual management of patients.

A Dream Come True

The Creation of the Queen Mother's Hospital

The concept of a new teaching maternity hospital for Glasgow had been in Donald's mind long before the building took its familiar shape on the skyline above the Yorkhill basin on Glasgow's famous River Clyde. He recounts that, at the time of his interview for the Regius Chair, he was asked what plans he might have for the future if he were to be appointed. Without hesitation he replied that he visualised a new modern maternity hospital in the west end of the city close to the University and the Western Infirmary and linked to the Royal Hospital for Sick Children.

His appointment to the Chair carried with it charge of a unit in the Glasgow Royal Maternity and Women's Hospital, known to generations of Glasgow women as "Rottenrow", but it was always in his mind that this was no more than a staging post until the hospital of his dreams materialised and with typical drive and enthusiasm he set about realising the dream.

His first objective was to find the money and there were two possible sources to be tapped. First was the Scottish Office, which was responsible for the allocation of government funds, and he harried them relentlessly until the promise of a sizeable contribution was secured. His other source was the university, since it was to be a teaching hospital and again he was success-ful, thanks in no small part to the influence of the Principal, Sir Hector Hetherington, who was much impressed by the personality and ambition of the new member of the senate.

The influence of the University was well illustrated at a crucial point in the planning process. The Western Regional Hospital Board had virtually decided that the new maternity hospital should be built in the north-east of Glasgow in the spacious grounds of Robroyston Hospital, formerly a tuberculosis sanatorium. At the meeting at which this was discussed, Sir Hector Hetherington was seen shuffling his papers, gently getting up, and was heard saying, in a quiet gentle voice, "You must excuse me, gentlemen, for you must know that if this proposal goes ahead, the University can have no further interest in the project. Good afternoon!". The Board reversed its decision at lightning speed because they knew that the university Principal was taking a vast sum of money away with him. He was prevailed upon to stay and the Yorkhill project went ahead.

Having thus obtained promises of the necessary funds, Ian Donald's next task was to find an architect who would put on paper the ideas (many of them revolutionary) that were brimming in his mind. In this he was indeed fortunate to secure the services of JL Gleave, whose youthful personality and enthusiasm dovetailed with that of Donald and, together, they produced a new design of maternity hospital which was to set aside many of the traditional patterns.

Hitherto, a maternity hospital consisted of two sets of wards, antenatal and postnatal, with a strict dichotomy between the two. The antenatal beds were for undelivered patients and most of these beds were occupied by the common complications of pregnancy, such as pre-eclampsia with raised blood pressure, swelling of the tissues and, in severe cases, culminating in convulsions, occasionally fatal to both mother and infant. In such cases, the fetal growth was often restricted, so that careful supervision and a prolonged stay in the antenatal ward were often required.

The remaining antenatal beds were usually occupied by patients being investigated and treated for antepartum haemorrhage or by those whose pregnancies were complicated by medical conditions such as diabetes or heart disease or renal disease.

The labour wards were usually communal, with such privacy as there was being provided by curtains. Normal and simple operative deliveries took place there. Women were only trans-ferred to the operating theatre for very complicated deliveries or for caesarean section.

The postnatal wards contained those women who were recovering from a normal delivery (it was usual for them to be retained in hospital for up to ten days) or from the effects of an operative or otherwise complicated delivery.

Donald's ideas changed all that.

The planned new hospital consisted of a central delivery block with separate nursing, medical and anaesthetic staff, and a separate delivery room for each woman and two operating theatres for caesarean sections and forceps or otherwise complicated deliveries.

From the central block there radiated four 'wings' designated North, South, West and East. The East wing, which had a separate room for each woman, was reserved for infected or seriously complicated cases. The beds in other wings were shared by the senior consultants, each of whom had his own junior staff. These wings contained small intimate four- or six-bedded wards and a number of single rooms. Antenatal and postnatal women were mixed together and the single rooms were reserved for those who required special antenatal or postnatal care.

At the far end of the hospital was the University Department containing a lecture room, a small library and the offices of the senior staff. This was surmounted by the Tower Block, containing living accommodation for the resident medical and nursing staff.

Construction of the hospital

The plans having finally been accepted, construction began in June 1960. Donald continued to be closely involved with each phase of the building. By some contrivance he managed to have appointed his own 'master of works', in the shape of Miss Marjory Marr, who had been his ward sister in Rottenrow and was later to become the first matron of the new hospital. As the building progressed, she was to be seen first prowling the foundations and later the development of each phase as it progressed. The workmen were cajoled and encouraged and amazed at her

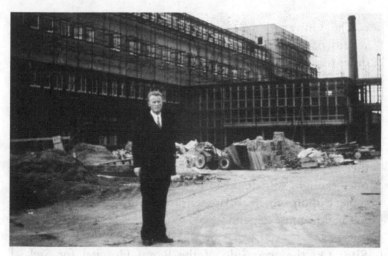

"Committee of One" – QMH building site

knowledge of basic building procedures. Each day she reported progress to the Professor and we are sure her activities contributed in no small measure to the speed with which the building rose.

By 1961, Ian Donald felt confident enough to write a detailed article for the "special series on hospital planning" published by the *Scottish Medical Journal*. Some quotations from this follow.

"The need for maternity hospital beds in Glasgow is acute. The housing shortage in the city and the inadequacy of much of the existing accommodation for domiciliary mid-wifery magnifies the problem so that the pressure on beds is not only on medical but on social grounds as well.
It is reckoned that the city requires an additional 240 beds. The new Maternity Hospital at Yorkhill is designated to provide 112 of these.

Furthermore, a properly equipped academic department of obstetrics is badly needed in order to bring under-graduate training up to date and to meet the still more rapidly growing needs of postgraduates.

The University of Glasgow has drastically altered the system of teaching midwifery to undergraduates and, in order to implement the new curriculum, which lays greater emphasis upon practical work and residence in hospital, the present teaching facilities must be urgently extended.

Present day clinical research requires far more facilities than of old when the analysis of simply portable specimens like blood, urine and faeces, in a biochemical laboratory tucked away in some unwanted corner of a backyard, was once thought sufficient to meet the scientific demands of a subject upon which so large a proportion of the health of the nation must depend.

Site: On the west side of the Royal Hospital for Sick Children there exists, fortunately, quite a large site which was once a hockey pitch. Many reasons determine the choice of this site. Firstly, the ground is immediately available, without the need for compulsory purchases, or demolitions. Secondly, its proximity to the Royal Hospital for Sick Children will provide a unique opportunity for collaboration with the staff of this hospital and the Institute of Child Health in meeting the problems of the newborn, whose importance now looms very large, especially since the hideous maternal mortality of a quarter of a century ago has been brought largely under control. Thirdly, such a hospital will be reasonably close to the University and to the Western Infirmary with its gynaecological department, which will be associated clinically with the new maternity hospital. The population on the west side of Glasgow and north of the Clyde is increasing very rapidly and is inadequately served at present in respect of maternity accommodation.

Lastly, by building within the grounds of an already existing hospital it is possible to reduce costs significantly in administration and, by common usage, in many of the existing facilities such as main kitchens, general stores, boiler heating and in maintenance, electrical and sanitary services. In the further application of this principle it is proposed to enlarge and extend the present departments of pathology, biochemistry and radiology to meet the needs of both hospitals together. Central sterilising and laundry services are also a likely economy. The site itself is impressive, standing on high ground overlooking the valley in the direction of Gilmorehill and the University to the north and the Clyde to the south and west with its docks, cranes and shipyards.

Labour ward and operating theatre suite: The greatest departure from conventional practice lies in this suite. The original design has been motivated by two fundamental principles, firstly to make normal labour as normal as possible both in its surroundings, atmosphere and technical trappings and, secondly, to treat all abnormalities with the punctiliousness of a surgical discipline. All operative procedures, even minor ones, such as low forceps delivery and perineal suture, will be undertaken only in the presence of full surgical facilities.

The common practice in obstetrical units throughout the country is to undertake forceps delivery, breech extractions, manual removal of the placenta and so forth in labour or delivery rooms commonly reserved for the second stage of labour, and to keep a special operating theatre in the background for the performance of abdominal operations, such as caesarean section.

For a long time it has appeared to the writer inappropriate to regard a forceps delivery as being in a different surgical category from, for example, caesarean section.

The risks of haemorrhage, shock, sepsis and the hazards to the baby are comparable in both and there would appear to be no very good reason for segregating these cases as being of a different surgical status. After all, one undertakes such trivial procedures as dilatation and curettage in gynaecological operating theatres with as much surgical respect as is accorded to a full-blown Manchester repair or hysterectomy, and it would seem illogical to repair a torn perineum in labour with less care than one would employ in colpoperineorrhaphy in gynaecological practice.

For this reason the labour ward suite is divided into two main but closely connected parts. Firstly, a series of normal delivery rooms, which are approached through what will be called the 'service corridor'. The patient will be free to walk in and out of one of these rooms allocated to her for her labour and across this corridor into a common first-stage lounge where she can remain ambulant in labour for as long as possible, view television and talk to her visitors and friends. Later, towards the end of the first stage when labour threatens to become more uncomfortable, she can retire to her room, there to be delivered by pupil midwives and students under the direction of the labour ward sisters and house surgeons, under conditions as closely as possible resembling the normality of her own home. Under these circumstances the patients' husbands will be able to visit their wives in labour without interfering with the surgical discipline of the suite as a whole.

If, however, labour becomes in any way abnormal, and some operative procedure has to be undertaken, the patient will be wheeled through a door, on the opposite side of her room, leading into what will be called the 'sterile' corridor.

She is now within the orbit of the theatre, throughout which full theatre disciplines will apply. This corridor opens into the suite of three main operating theatres, staffed by a regular theatre staff and maintaining a 24 hours service. One of these theatres will be reserved for major obstetrical operations, but the other two will be used for the more standard and everyday procedures.

It is expected that these theatres will be in constant use and at a constant pitch of efficiency and great economy in time, effort and expense should be achieved. The completely normal case will never see the inside of this suite and will get no further than her own little delivery room, which will have none of the surgical atmosphere so terrifying to many patients. But all surgical procedures, both major and minor, will be carried out under the best possible surgical conditions.

It will be possible to look down into the theatres through slanting glass walls, separating the theatre from the galleries above. Microphonic communication will connect the two and because these galleries will be above and beyond the lighting over the operating tables it will be possible to observe what is going on below without being seen. This will be very useful for both students and doctors who will be able to take stock of the situation without the need for changing and washing before coming down into the theatre proper, should this be necessary. This will limit unnecessary coming and going into the theatre and will reduce infection.

The future: Every battleship, at its launch, is reputed to be already out of date. None of us has the gift of prophecy and it is difficult to foretell the likely changes which will take place in obstetrics, but to the best of our knowledge it is reasonably clear that the institutional delivery rate will rise and that the public, who are compulsory subscribers to the National Health Service, will increasingly demand hospital confinement. Domiciliary delivery has practically died already in Australia, Sweden and in much of the United States. It is also clear that the operative delivery rate will rise. Normal labour is all very well and to be encouraged, but it can be secured at too great a price in effort and suffering. For a woman to push for two hours in the second stage with the head low in the pelvis in the hope of securing a spontaneous vaginal delivery is now nothing more than a barbaric anachronism.

The present day perinatal mortality rate, which has not shown much improvement over many years, is a matter of the greatest concern and hospital facilities must be increasingly directed towards providing the means to reduce it.

Research may presently put within our grasp methods of controlling intra-uterine development and of estimating and improving placental function in order to forestall intrauterine fetal death and macerated stillbirth to reduce the incidence of prematurity and to secure the delivery of babies far healthier at birth. These exciting possibilities may put a different but none the less important emphasis upon the need for antenatal beds. With the policy in this hospital of being able to interchange the functions of antenatal and lying-in beds it is hoped to be able to meet the foreseeable changes in obstetric practice.

In this age of rapid medical progress modern hospitals face obsolescence within 25 years of their completion.

This is a sobering thought and lays heavy responsibility upon those of us concerned with the planning of a new hospital such as this, but the spirit of co-operating and enthusiasm with which everyone concerned with this project has infused and infected his colleagues must surely go a long way in securing for the City and its University a unit as good as the wit of man can at present devise".

Equipping

Having ensured that the building was complete Donald then devoted himself to equipping the hospital and each day he was to be seen poring over schedules and deciding on the items of equipment which would be required, down to the last item of furniture and the last instrument in the operating theatre. We particularly remember being asked how many spare coat hangers would be required in our offices. Frequent planning meetings were held in the unfinished hospital. We remember struggling up incomplete brickwork stairs with inadequate lighting. There was a thrill about this because at the next meeting there were signs of progress in the building.

Donald introduced several other measures, which, at that time, were considered revolutionary. Patient visiting was allowed at any time of the day as long as it did not interfere with the normal running of the ward, and there was no restriction on the number of visitors at each bed. This was indeed a radical change from the existing hospital practice of having set visiting hours heralded by the clanging of a bell and a rush of friends and relations clutching the traditional bunch of flowers and bottle of Lucozade, all to be dismissed by another clang of the bell at the end of two hours.

It was also at about this time that the practice of allowing husbands to be present at delivery was introduced. Donald, with his strict upbringing, was not enthusiastic about the idea, but permitted it nonetheless.

He also introduced a new records system. Each woman, on being referred to the hospital antenatal clinic, was allocated a coloured disc which was attached to all her documents and attached her to a consultant who, with his team, would be responsible for her management throughout the pregnancy. She would attend his clinic and be housed in his wing and be supervised by him and his junior staff. In this way, the woman identified with a particular consultant and this gave her a sense of belonging to a team. In our opinion, this is preferable to the modern practice of a woman not knowing who is responsible for her care or her delivery. In many cases she is often sent home so soon after delivery that she has no idea who was her obstetrician.

Another innovation introduced at this time was the holding of a weekly perinatal conference. This was attended not only by the medical and nursing staff of the hospital but also by representatives from the Royal Hospital for Sick Children who were responsible for the resuscitation of infants after birth. There were also members of the pathology department and the anaesthetic department who all contributed at appropriate times. Particular care was given to any perinatal loss and these discussions not only helped to elucidate the facts and suggest any possible future changes but, most of all, they promoted the feeling of partnership and cooperation between members of the various disciplines.

The canteen was situated centrally in the hospital and Donald insisted that there should be no tables set aside for special groups such as consultant or senior nursing staff. It was hoped by him that there should be a complete mix of staff and he made a point of sitting with cleaners, porters and junior nurses. It was one of his ideas that really did not succeed and, within a few weeks, the various groups of nurses, doctors and so on, had gravitated towards their own kind.

Public interest in the construction of the new hospital was considerable and the newspapers kept the public well informed. On 13th September 1962, the *Evening Times* reported, "Good progress is being made on the new £800,000 maternity hospital being built at Yorkhill, Glasgow. The architect for the hospital, Mr JL Gleave, said:'In spite of the weather we have had, the main contractors, Crudens Ltd, are up to date in their work'. Accommodation for 112 patients will be provided at the hospital, which will be the first of its kind to use an ultrasonic echo-sounding technique developed at the Western Infirmary to help in diagnosing the early stages of pregnancy". Another newspaper report on 9th January 1964, stated, "Glasgow's first complete, all new hospital since the beginning of World War II will have its first patients on Saturday". Ian Donald was keen to get the unit going as early as was safe, so, symbolically, we entered an incomplete building to convey the idea that the builders had better get a move on. Only twenty-four of the 114 beds were ready but a beginning was made and there were no medical disasters. The first woman to give birth in the hospital, Mrs Mavis Rennie, was lyrical about the facilities and remained a keen supporter of Professor Donald until he retired.

Before the hospital opened officially, the journalist Deirdre Chapman also gave birth there. She was just as enthusiastic as Mrs Rennie and wrote in *The Express*,

At 3.00 am one August morning, tucked into bed with a television set, radio, and magazine, it hit me that finally life was better with the National Health Service. For you can't buy your way into this hospital. There are no private patients. It is run like a four-star holiday camp. Gone is the 'left-along-for-two-hours-in-a-draughty-corridor' stage of labour. This is passed in a private First Stage Lounge. The journey from there to the labour room is accomplished in bed, without being manhandled on to a trolley. And if you have to go into the operating theatre, the inevitable flock of students watches from a hidden gallery – mercifully from both the sterile and the social point of view. When you arrive in a four-bed ward or a single room (you have the choice) you realise that there are no rules at all. "If I catch anyone giving an order, I cancel it", said Professor Ian Donald, the senior consultant with a twinkle. "I won't have any notices saying 'No Smoking' or 'The Visiting Hours Are . . .'. Our intention is to treat patients as humanly as possible.

So, there is feeding on demand, afternoon AND evening visiting, and life resolves itself into a series of languid decisions . . . Shall I have a bath or a shower? Shall I feed the baby now or after lunch? Will I have tea or coffee. The babies, by the way, live alongside their mothers in a sort of stainless steel trolley. The laundry stays in a cupboard underneath. The responsibility for it is all yours. To feed baby, you shut yourself off from the world in a tent of chintzy patterns. Visitors who arrive meanwhile wait for you in the luxurious glass-walled lounge adjoining the ward. You totter out 20 minutes later to join them, feeling rather indecent in limp quilted nylon, and look around automatically for the waiter to order drinks. When the doctors do their round you will very probably miss them, for there is no "Hush, hush, here comes matron" attitude about staying in bed."

At first the sumptuousness of it all can be a little trying. But soon you become proud at being a pioneer of new-deal childbirth in the most modern maternity hospital in Britain.

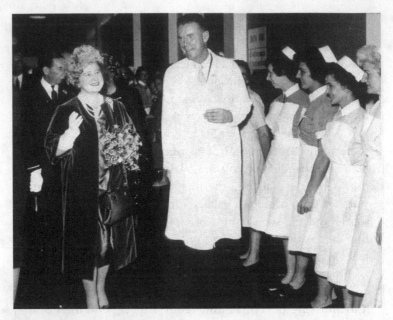

The Queen Mother opening QMH

The official opening by Her Majesty Queen Elizabeth the Queen Mother took place on 23rd September 1964. In addition to performing her official duties with customary grace, she showed a keen interest in the hospital, about which she was already well informed, and asked Professor Donald some searching questions as she went around. There was a tense moment when she insisted on seeing the viewing gallery above the operating theatre, not on the official itinerary. It was reached by a narrow spiral stair and there was panic when some people imagined that there would be an accident with her very narrow high-heeled shoes. But she was up and down the stairs like a chamois and all was well.

In her official speech, the Queen Mother described the hospital as, "unique in being combined with a children's hospital, thus giving care where needed to the newborn baby, infant and growing child. That this hospital is also linked with the University of Glasgow, is, I feel an important step not only in the interests of teaching, upon which a new generation of doctors will depend, but also in the interests of research upon which may be founded fresh advances and knowledge". Addressing the nursing staff, the Queen Mother said they held the key to making it a really good hospital and ensuring the happiness of the patients. They could share with a family, she said, in the most wonderful happiness in the world, the birth of a child.

It was all in all a wonderful day. "Bliss was it in that dawn to be alive". However, it was time to get down to work. The consultant staff were Professor Ian Donald, Drs McBride, Barr, MacVicar and Willocks.

Ian McBride has not been mentioned before in this narrative, but he was a powerful force in the Queen Mother's Hospital. After wartime service in the RAF, where he had a distinguished career taking part in the invasion of Crete, he joined Professor RA Lennie as Assistant Obstetric Surgeon (as they were called in these days) at Glasgow Royal Maternity Hospital. At the Royal Samaritan (gynaecological) Hospital he did some important work on endometrial carcinoma. Ian McBride was direct, plain speaking and supremely honest. As such, he certainly did not please everyone. A superb clinical teacher, he was known by the junior staff as "The Master" and brought this name to the Queen Mother's Hospital. Ian Donald and Ian McBride had been colleagues for ten years when the Queen Mother's Hospital opened. There were doubts about whether he would join the new hospital and the Professor approached him in an off-hand way and asked "Would you like to come to the new hospital?". To which the reply was "Would you like to have me in the new hospital?"; the reply was a subdued affirmative. A vibrant, humorous personality, Ian McBride plunged himself into the new hospital with tremendous energy and was greatly loved by the junior staff. When they wanted him he was there (as indeed we all were) but he was liable to telephone a registrar or house surgeon at 7.30 a.m. and ask "What are you doing about Mrs So-and-So? She has a problem" and put down the telephone because he had already solved the problem. Later, he became the first RCOG Regional Postgraduate Adviser for the West of Scotland (a vast area in which he knew personally all the senior staff and helped the juniors enormously). His description of postgraduate training was succinct:

1. You assist me.
2. I assist you.
3. You do it unsupervised.
4. You decide what is to be done.

How different is the bureaucratic postgraduate mechanism today!

Ian McBride retired at the age of sixty years and moved to Easingwold, Yorkshire. He became a history student at the University of York, with special interest in nineteenth-century France, ending as an expert on such characters as Victor Hugo and his arch-enemy 'Napoleon le Petit' (Napoleon III). This was an innovative way to spend one's retirement. He later developed Parkinson's disease, moved back to Glasgow, and died in 1996.

Registrars and house officers who became professors and consultants in later life abounded. Being adjacent to the Royal Hospital for Sick Children, full paediatric facilities were available and Professor James Hutchison was keen to provide them. Special mention must be made of Dr Margaret Kerr, neonatologist, whose devotion to saving premature or ill babies was unbounded.

The Consultant Anaesthetist was Donald Moir, a pupil of Robert Hingson, the American inventor of epidural anaesthesia. Dr Moir used it in the Queen Mother's Hospital with Ian Donald's support and continuous lumbar epidural analgesia was used in 146 patients in 1964–65.

Full laboratory services were available and mention must be made of Michael Willoughby, Consultant Haematologist, who introduced iron and folic acid supplements for antenatal patients with enormous benefit to anaemic women in Glasgow.

The cardiologist, Alister Cameron, was Ian Donald's adviser before his first operation and ran a busy clinic, rheumatic heart disease in women being common at that time.

The Matron of the hospital was Miss Marjorie E Marr, who had been Professor Donald's ward sister in Rottenrow and who knew his ways well. She had been involved in the planning and building of the new hospital and captained a very efficient nursing ship. We remember the keenness and efficiency of ward sisters and nurses from the beginning.

The first clinical report for 1964–65 states in its preface "The Queen Mother's Hospital did not spring like Minerva from the head of Jove, armed at all points, but serious clinical work began even before the building was complete and detailed case records were kept from the start. We owe a great debt to the cheerful efficiency of the Medical Records Officer, Mr Robert Ferguson, and his staff. We are grateful to all our medical and nursing colleagues who have helped in the collection of information, particularly Dr Andrew Sarbah-Yalley,[2] who did a great deal of work in the final stages". It was really a team effort, with people working willingly out of hours. The total number of births in this period was 4,767. The number of antenatal attendances was 31,395 and postnatal attendances 2,799. The number of attendances at the cardiac clinic was 1,040, seventy-two percent of women had completely normal births and the caesarean section rate was 7.1 percent. Ultrasonic examinations were not classified separately in this report, but by 1970–71, there were 4,119 examinations on Queen Mother's Hospital patients and 878 on patients from other hospitals. Clinically, it was a busy unit from the start. All medical staff had full clinical responsibilities and research was done in their spare time. In heading the hospital of his creation Ian Donald at first behaved as a 'Grand Monarch', conducting rounds of the whole hospital in the manner of the Saturday morning rounds in the Western Infirmary.

---

2 Andrew Sarbah-Yalley BSc MD FRCOG from Accra, Ghana was a genial colleague and became eminent as a teacher in the Korle Bu Teaching Hospital. Being from an aristocratic family, he inherited a title and became a Prince, or as we would say in Scotland, a clan chief.

This method proved unsatisfactory, due to the vast numbers of clinical problems to be discussed and, on the instigation of Ian McBride, each of the consultants (including the Professor) became responsible for his own clinic and patients. This was much more practical. There were frequent meetings, professional and social; indeed, the consultants met every day and clinical problems were freely discussed. It was a very friendly atmosphere with lots of wit and humour among us.

A very important figure in Ian Donald's life was Miss Adèle Ure, his secretary. Formerly secretary to Professor Lennie at Rottenrow, Ian knew her from his arrival in Glasgow and depended upon her increasingly. Gentle, ladylike and unflappable she took everything in her stride, be it mountains of typing, arrangements for exams and visitors and organising foreign trips. She was a calming and de-stressing influence and he could not have done without her.

The new hospital was envied throughout the United Kingdom and visitors were frequent. Alistair Miller recounts, "Ian Donald's pride in his hospital was enormous – 'every woman a Duchess!'. I remember an early visit from Chassar Moir, Bill Hawksworth and John Stallworthy (what a trio!) who were planning the new John Radcliffe Maternity Hospital in Oxford. We did a forceps delivery for them with Ian Donald providing a continuous commentary to the gallery". The Oxford team went away with new ideas, which they incorporated in the new building. Alistair Miller also writes, "Attracting Donald Moir (anaesthetist) and Michael Willoughby (haematologist) to provide new services showed Ian Donald's foresight. I remember an encounter between him and Michael during a ward round in the West Wing. We were studying a haematology report when Michael came in to see another patient. Ian Donald at once hailed him and, towering over him, said 'Michael, tell me are the terms macrocyte and megaloblast interchangeable?' Michael paused for a moment, rocking on his heels, one hand cupping his elbow and replied, 'For you, yes'. The other point I always remember, thinking of the present problems of the hospital is that, although Ian Donald loved it, he used to say, 'Of course, this place is Jerry-built. It will fall down in 30 years'. Too near the truth unhappily."

We think that Ian Donald recognised that from the beginning, even at the planning stage. We think he would have approved of Sir James Simpson's point of view in the nineteenth century that hospitals should be disposable, to prevent infection and allow modern improvements.

Ultrasound was of prime importance in Ian Donald's mind in the new hospital with its increased facilities for diagnosis (a change from the primitive A-scope machine which was all that was available in Rottenrow) and he viewed the technique as his personal property for clinical research even in the labour ward.

Again, Alistair Miller recounts an experience from 1966. "I was the registrar on call and Ian Donald came up to say that if I had a forceps delivery to be done under general anaesthesia (not uncommon even though we had started with epidurals) he wanted to be called as he wished to try to locate the placenta by ultrasound. A suitable case duly arrived later in the day. An ultrasound machine appeared (still very large) in theatre. I delivered the baby. No oxytocic drug was given and I then determined the position of the placenta on the uterine wall. Ian Donald took repeated films (as we allowed the third stage of labour to proceed naturally) and I checked the position of the placenta as it descended in the birth canal. At the end of it all, he was quite unable to identify the placenta on the films and was very despondent."

Less than two years later Alistair was back from his spell in Nairobi, at the Kenyatta Hospital where Glasgow University supported the new maternity unit under the direction of John MacVicar. There was no diagnostic ultrasound there, of course. "It was Monday morning and I had just completed my first weekend on call. We would report on the weekend's events to Ian Donald before he embarked on his marathon round of the whole hospital. I had delivered successfully by caesarean section a baby with a prolapsed cord and thought I might get some praise, remembering his textbook comment about 'a landmark in a young obstetrician's life' when he saved his first baby with cord prolapse. No praise was forthcoming. He was more interested in a case of undiagnosed twins which I had suspected and sent for confirmation by X-ray. Before leaving he asked me to go to his room at the end of the round. I'm afraid the penny did not drop even then. He said on my preference for X-ray over ultrasound 'Alistair, you either didn't think of using ultrasound to confirm the twins, or you thought of it and rejected it in favour of an X-ray'. I said that I had just returned from Kenya and did not realise how much more ultrasound was being used in Glasgow. I don't think he was convinced. On ultrasound, as with other innovations, his imagination always ran ahead to some new possibility. In the late 1960s, he talked about measuring the thickness of the placenta as an indication of the severity of rhesus disease. That didn't happen of course, but the study of placental texture has come about similarly when he was looking at high and low implantations of the gestation sac with Andrew Yalley. We were all getting sceptical but I suppose this did lead the way to crown–rump length of the fetus as an indication of development."

Ian Donald viewed ultrasound as his personal province and strove to win new triumphs. Like St Paul (one of his favourite authors) who wrote, "This one thing I do, forgetting those things which are behind, and reaching forth unto those things which are before, I press towards the mark for the prize". But he could not be everywhere, especially in later years. He was fortunate in acquiring a personal assistant in the ultrasonic department. Mrs Ida Miller was the wife of Ian Donald's general practitioner. Intelligent and decisive, she quickly acquired scanning skills and was directed by the Professor from his office with closed circuit television. Thus, Ian Donald, like an actor-manager of the old school, continued to direct the productions and play the principal parts himself.

Looking back on it, the first ten years of the Queen Mother's Hospital were golden years. A study of Glasgow births in 1963 just before the new hospital opened, showed a hospital birth rate of seventy percent but concluded that ninety percent of women had an acceptable indication for hospital birth. The study went on to say that the selection of cases for hospital delivery was inefficient. Of first births, ten percent were not delivered in hospital and the figure for those having their fourth or later children was forty percent. During the ten years 1963–73, the situation changed radically and the Queen Mother's Hospital played its part in this, making 2,100 bookings annually on a medical basis and leaving 400 places for emergency cases and socially disadvantaged patients.

Our main objective was quite simple, to put the woman first, inspiring confidence, always addressing her by name and giving a clear explanation of what was happening to her and never leaving her alone for any length of time during labour. Frequent antenatal visits resulted in familiarity with the staff who were looking after her and diminished her fear. The same consultant and registrar who saw her at the clinic were responsible for her management during labour. Every attempt was made to make decisions at the antenatal clinic so that wasteful and unnecessary admissions might be avoided and the woman was not left in uncertainty, following the maxim "The good doctor may not have made a diagnosis but he has made a decision: the bad doctor has made neither". That is how we saw it in the mid 1970s and certainly things worked well.

When Professor Donald retired in 1976, his successor was Professor Charles Whitfield, who was the first postgraduate student at the hospital in 1964. He carried on the traditions and infused new ideas. But that is another story.

SCIENCE AND SERENDIPITY
The Birth of Medical Ultrasound

"A man that looks on glass
On it may stay his eye
Or if he pleaseth through it pass
And then the heavens espy."

These lines by the seventeenth-century poet George Herbert convey the role of imagination in research. They were used by Ian Donald to introduce his Victor Bonney lecture delivered to the Royal College of Surgeons of England on 31st October 1973, which is one of the many accounts given by him over the years describing the development of medical ultrasound. Its title is "Apologia"– not an expression of regret, but a spirited self-defence. (He added that he hoped its consequences would not be as lethal for the author as Socrates' "Apologia" was for him.)

Ian believed that accident and good luck had combined at the right time to open up for the medical profession a new diagnostic dimension. In the experiment, most of the worthwhile observations were unforeseen. A similar attitude was shown by Max Perutz, who won the Nobel Prize for his discovery of the structure of haemoglobin. "Creativity in science, as in the arts, cannot be organised. It arises spontaneously from individual talent. Well-run laboratories can foster it, but hierarchical organisation, inflexible, bureaucratic rules and mountains of futile paperwork can kill it. Discoveries cannot be planned; they pop up, like Puck, in unexpected corners."

With the present bureaucratic 'evidence based' attitude to medicine, where multiple criteria have to be fulfilled before doing anything, it is doubtful whether Ian's experiment would have got off the ground, but he says he was driven inexorably onwards, so the bureaucrats would have a lot to battle with if he were alive today!

The early days of ultrasound are vividly recalled by Ian in an address given to medical students in 1965. He was a seeker of the truth, but also a tireless self-publicist. Out of the many lectures he gave, we have selected what we think are the most readable extracts. One of these turned-up unexpectedly in the *British Journal of Non-Destructive Testing* in 1992 and is a reprint of a talk delivered to a student audience in 1965.

"I had not given much thought to the subject of ultrasonic echo sounding as a diagnostic method before my relocation from London to Glasgow ten years ago. Indeed, at that time my knowledge was limited to the sort of general knowledge possessed by most of us. Every boy of my generation knew about ASDIC (the word stands for 'Anti-Submarine Detection and Investigation Committee'), which was developed by using echo sounding for locating U-boats towards the end of the 1914–18 War, when this committee was set up jointly by the French and British Admiralties to meet the terrible menace of the German submarine campaign. During the 1920s, I had read of and seen demonstrations of charting the ocean bed, again by echo sounding. During my years in the Royal Air Force in the last War I had become familiar with a variety of radar techniques and had developed a hearty respect for what electronic science could do. Since my time was spent almost wholly with operational squadrons engaged on highly secret work, again fighting the German U-boat menace, I flew a bit with the crews in our heavy four-engine bombers and, on the ground, took a good deal of interest in the various activities that were going on in the flight offices and various technical sections of the large aerodromes to which I was attached. In those days, miniaturised or micro methods of echo sounding had not come into use for detecting flaws in metal structures, for example in the main spar of an aircraft wing, and one had to rely on signs of paint wrinkling on the surface of a spar to be warned of underlying metal fatigue.

I recall one crash in which part of an aeroplane's wing broke off with the death of all the occupants and it was averred that this type of inspection had not been properly carried out in time to prevent such an accident.

Ultrasonic techniques for medical diagnosis were first attempted in the late 1940s by Dussik in Austria without very encouraging success but in the early 1950s echo sounding methods, as used in the detection of flaws in metals, began to look a little more promising. I was vaguely aware of some of this work being attempted in the United States and, in fact, had been visited one afternoon by one of the pioneers from Minneapolis, namely Wild. He was trying to see if there were different echo characteristics between a lump in the breast which was benign and one which was malignant. This approach did not capture the imagination of the average surgeon, since none would rely on such investigation or be content with anything less than biopsy.

It was against this background that I more or less inadvertently drifted into the subject in 1955, some months after I had arrived in Glasgow.[1]

It happened that I was lent an ultrasonic generator by a friend of a friend in a scientific instrument factory near Paisley and in my then ignorance I had the idea of

---

1 WB recollects that he was there at the moment of the conception of diagnostic ultrasound in gynaecology. When Ian Donald came to Glasgow WB was his fellow consultant at the Western Infirmary and it was their custom, when finished work, to review the events of the day over a glass of sherry. Ian was looking for a fresh research project. One day he came in and said "I think I've found it!" and proceeded to produce an article about submarine detection. He said "I think this ASDIC technique could be applied to medicine," and the next thing was that he had to find a suitable detector.

generating a frequency sufficiently high to shatter cells by means of resonance.

I started by trying to haemolise blood. This was easy enough at high energies but I noticed that the degree of haemolysis depended directly upon the amount of heat generated in the solution under test and, in fact, parallel experiments at controlled temperature yielded exactly the same degree of haemolysis. Professor Feather at the University of Edinburgh put me in touch with a certain amount of literature on the subject and I soon learned that this kind of thing had already been done in the United States as a means of producing experimental destructive lesions in the central nervous system in animals. At about this time, high-power ultrasound of this type was employed to inflict prefrontal leucotomy on humans but, as far as could be seen, the effects again were inseparable from those due to locally generated heat. Any hope I had of destroying the relatively large nuclei of malignant cells differentially from surrounding tissues with smaller nuclei began quickly to evaporate as I learned of German attempts at this with uniformly depressing results.

In my early attempts to acquire some knowledge of this subject of ultrasound, however, I had read and very fully digested an excellent textbook on ultrasonics by Carlin and my interest turned to very low energy and refined echo sounding techniques employed in metals in industry. This was clearly an altogether different subject from the destructive effects of high powered ultrasound and by a piece of sheer good fortune, and through a patient on whom I had successfully operated, I got an introduction to the research department of a large engineering firm in Renfrew, Messrs Babcock and Wilcox, who build boilers for atomic power stations and who I heard were using ultrasonic echo sounding to detect any flaws in their boiler welds. I was invited to meet the directors of this research department and I can remember they stood me a very good lunch at Renfrew Airport.

The upshot of this friendly meeting was that it was agreed that we [ID and WB] would bring down to them on the following Friday afternoon a number of tumours recently excised and they would use their flaw detecting instruments to see if different types of tumours, for example ovarian cysts, had different echo characteristics from solid tumours such as uterine fibroids.

Accordingly the best tumours from our 'waiting list' were got into hospital and were duly removed from their owners a day or so before, and then loaded into the boots of two cars and we set off to Renfrew.

On arrival, we found that our industrial friends had provided an enormous lump of steak to act as a control material. Behind closed doors, since the experiment to the lay mind lacked a certain amount of elegance, we used their metal flaw detecting probes on the specimens of ovarian cysts and fibroids and the lump of steak, and to my great excitement it was clear that different echoes were produced by different types of tumour. It was difficult to interpret the information which appeared on their cathode ray tubes but of the differences there could be no doubt, and the experiment seemed to be repeatable. At the end of this highly profitable afternoon there was some dispute as to who should take charge of the steak and I am sorry to say that nobody seemed to want it!

It was agreed that I should borrow one of their flaw detectors and I decided that I would confine my investigations to clinically obvious tumours to see if I could reproduce in vivo what had been done at the research department of the boiler factory. To examine a human abdomen with its multiplicity of different tissues all in unpredictable positions and levels is quite another and our first experiments were very disappointing.

Our friends in the boiler factory began to get possibly a little tired of lending us equipment and suggested putting us in touch with the makers of their flaw detectors, namely

Messrs Kelvin and Hughes, who were also situated not too far away in the Hillington Factory Estate near Renfrew Airport. As luck would have it, I happened to be in the process of selling a sailing boat to one of the public relations officers of this firm and he introduced me to the directors, who expressed a wish to meet me and accordingly I invited them to lunch at the Western Infirmary and explained to them what I was trying to do. I also demonstrated the kind of echoes one could get from a large ovarian cyst in a water tank. These three directors took a very sporting view of the experiment and decided to vote a certain limited sum towards these experiments (I believe £500). That was in 1955, since when expenditure has run well into five figures. I was thus lent a Kelvin and Hughes Mark IV flaw detector, which in its day was the most advanced machine of its sort.

So far we had found that using a hand-held probe and directing an ultrasonic beam into an abdomen, echoes from intestine lying underneath the abdominal wall were all crowded up at close range and were very strong and 'dancing'. But if there was a large quantity of fluid, for example an ovarian cyst, which kept these strong echoes from the bowel out of the way, there was a clear gap until the other side of the cyst was reached. We immediately tried to distinguish between ascites (free fluid in the abdomen) and an ovarian cyst because, in an ovarian cyst, the echoes from intestine are pushed to one side, whereas in ascites the bowel floats up under the abdominal wall close to the probe and produces the echoes at closer range. Conversely, in ascites the flanks form troughs of fluid, which are responsible for the well-known physical sign of shifting dullness and produce a separation between probe and bowel echoes in this site.

Our first difficulties were to make contact between the probe and the patient. We did this initially by using a plastic bucket of about 8 cm in diameter with a latex rubber bottom, which we filled with water. This was then balanced precariously on top of the patient's abdomen, which had first been smeared with lubricating jelly, so as to eliminate air pockets. The probe was then dipped gingerly into the surface of the water and undignified accidents were frequent. We later learned to apply the probe direct to the abdominal skin using a coupling film of olive oil. The basis of echo sounding is really quite simple and depends upon the fact that sound will travel through a homogeneous substance at a standard velocity, but when it encounters some substance of different physical properties some of the energy at the boundary between the two tissues is in specific acoustic impedance (specific acoustic impedance, i.e. the product of the density and the velocity of the sound wave within it). It is for this reason that bowel which contains gas of very low density, compared with tissue, sends back such powerful echoes. Theoretically one would expect a fairly homogeneous structure like a fibroid to attenuate the ultrasound in its passage through it, while an ovarian cyst, being full of clear fluid, would inflict no such attenuation. We reckoned that whereas there would be little residual energy left to produce an echo from the far side of a fibroid, the far wall of an ovarian cyst would be able to send back strong echoes and this we found to be the case. I need not be reminded that one can tell the difference between an ovarian cyst and a fibroid on clinical grounds, but that was not the important point. It was necessary to start from humble beginnings in order to get down to more refined techniques.

It was about this time that we had the biggest stroke of beginners' luck. Colleagues in Professor Wayne's Department of Medicine had heard of our interest in demonstrating ascites and invited me to use our flaw detector on a patient in their wards who was reputed to be dying from a carcinoma of the stomach with portal obstruction and ascites. She was vomiting and losing weight rapidly and a barium X-ray supported the diagnosis. Clinically, the patient, a middle-aged woman, had an extremely tense abdomen and, as often happens in such cases, the physical signs were deceptive.

I agreed with the diagnosis of ascites and applied the probe to the abdominal wall whereupon, to my dismay, I observed a long clear gap and strong echoes only at depth (having expected echoes from bowel close under the abdominal wall). At this moment, my colleague, Dr MacVicar, looked over the screen and, not knowing anything of the background, commented, "It looks like a cyst". I was in the process of apologising to the bystanders for the failure of the experiment since the suggestion of a cyst seemed preposterous. However, it was agreed to demonstrate the case at a forthcoming Tuesday evening forum at the Western Infirmary and the same ultrasonic findings were manifested. It then appeared that the physicians were by no means committed to the diagnosis of portal obstruction and ascites, and it was agreed that I would be allowed to operate. Some days later at laparotomy, to my wild surprise and great delight, I found an enormous pseudomucinous cyst of the ovary completely filling the abdomen and which was histologically benign. The patient thereafter made a complete recovery, all vomiting and haematemesis ceased and for some years afterwards I was inflicted with horrid specimens of her grandchild's attempts at cooking by way of an expression of gratitude. There can be no doubt that this woman owed her survival to the ultrasonic findings which first cast doubt on what had appeared a clear diagnosis.

From this point onwards both I and the directors of Kelvin and Hughes, in particular Mr Slater, who has seen this project right through all these years, were determined to press on. So far, our experiments had been entirely confined to unidimensional, or A-scope presentation, that is to say we could detect echoes and estimate their strength by seeing vertical 'blips' on the horizontal time base of a cathode ray tube, but it was often difficult to make sense of so many echoes which were presented by all the tissue planes and interfaces of the body through which the ultrasonic beam might be passing.

We learned from Chowry's studies in the USA that an echo would only return to the probe and be recorded if the ultrasonic beam struck the reflecting interface or surface at right angles, since the laws of incidence and reflection apply, as in the case of light. What was really wanted was a technique which would map the position of these echoes in at least two dimensions. At this point one of the then junior electronic engineers in Messrs Kelvin and Hughes, Mr Tom Brown, came on the scene and offered help.

We agreed that some method of scanning was necessary and were already aware of the B-scan methods used in America and Japan, which produce a two-dimensional display of sorts and in which the probe moves in the plane of the section under review and plots the echoes as dots of light from any surface which happens to be at right angles to the incident ultrasonic beam. Because of the different angles of tilt of reflecting interfaces in the body which are unpredictable, we decided to use a rotating compound scanning search technique, rather like the sector scanning of radar, in order to increase the amount of echo information available and thus displayed on a cathode ray tube. A camera with an open shutter placed in front of this tube then recorded the position of all these echoes as they were picked up by the scanning probe.

The first compound scanning machine was fairly crude but at least we got pictures of a sort. The camera was an ordinary affair and we had to develop the films there and then, which was extremely tiresome, but the use of a Polaroid camera with almost instantaneous development of the pictures soon accelerated progress.[1]

---

1 Ian Donald soon showed typical impatience with the Polaroid camera, fuming and complaining, "Two minutes is far too long!".

We found that it was possible not only to outline an ovarian cyst, but to show up fetal echoes in a pregnant uterus and to outline the greater part of a baby's head.

We also found that our original theories about ascites and the echoes we would get from them were correct and, what was even more interesting, that when the ascites was due to peritoneal carcinomatosis, a much more bizarre picture was produced because the fluid in such cases surrounded masses of growth and intestine adherent to infiltrated omentum and so forth. The picture is so characteristic that the diagnosis can be made at once. We now went to press in a big way in 1958 and I produced the first major article with Dr MacVicar and Mr Brown as co-authors in *The Lancet*. In this article, the physics of our experiment is described more fully than I have ever since bothered to outline it in subsequent publications, especially as I have had more to say and relatively less space in which to say it as time has gone on.

At this period, between 1958 and 1959, I began to get worried about producing artefacts from scanning deliberately so as to 'sit on' echoes appearing on the monitoring tubes, mainly from fear of missing them. This was indeed a real fear and I can remember periods of as long as three weeks at a stretch without being able to produce a decent diagnostic picture in those days, whereas now I am really put out if we do not get at least some intelligible information out of every case investigated.

I, therefore, asked Messrs Kelvin and Hughes for an apparatus which automatically scanned the surface of the abdomen at a standard rate and rocking speed. As a result of this, a very complicated, but beautifully engineered, auto-matic scanner was produced which is pressure sensitive and will climb up hill and down dale over the contours of the patient's abdomen at a standard pressure and traversing it at standard speed.

This scanning apparatus is now installed in the X-ray

department at the Western Infirmary and has done nearly five years' yeoman service. Unfortunately, it produces a number of complications from electrical interference due to the switching on and off of the driving and reversing motors and in our newest models we have dispensed with this expensive mechanism. Nevertheless, it was necessary for a time in order to eliminate artefacts and from now on a very great experience was obtained.

The whole project was becoming so expensive that Messrs Kelvin and Hughes expressed a desire to pull out, although they agreed to complete the present automatic scanning machine and I could see the whole research project coming to a painful stop for lack of funds. The running costs were met by my research grant from the Scottish Hospital Endowments Trust, but it did not run to providing capital equipment costing many thousands of pounds to construct. I consulted the late Sir Hector Hetherington, then Principal of the University, and he immediately produced £750 to shore up the project temporarily while I sought help from the Scottish Hospital Endowments Research Trust and the Department of Health for Scotland. The Trust immediately came to my aid with a straight grant of £4000 and sent me onto the National Research Development Corporation in London where a further £10,000 to commission the building of new apparatus was finally arranged. This helped to quell the very natural alarm at the way in which money was being run away with at Messrs Kelvin and Hughes. Fortunately, about this time a merger with S Smith & Sons (England) Ltd, which is a very large concern with a considerable diversification of industrial interests, took place and the ultrasonic projects of Kelvin and Hughes became absorbed into a larger organisation which has so far continued to support the project. I would like here and now to express my gratitude to my friends in Kelvin and Hughes and latterly Smiths for their continued support, without which we could not have got as far as we have, and to the Scottish Hospital Endowment Research Trust.

In the meantime we scanned many hundreds and hundreds of cases, both pregnant and not pregnant, and our work has been punctuated by the occasional brainwave. I have already mentioned the distinction between malignant and nonmalignant ascites and the different pictures which are characteristic. We found that fetal echoes were demonstrable at a fairly early stage and this led on to the distinction between a case of threatened abortion with bleeding and a case of hydatidiform mole, also with bleeding, since the latter produces a curious, speckled picture, as might be expected, whereas a fetus produces clear strong echoes floating in a space containing liquor. As one result of this discovery we began to get a large number of cases referred to us for this particular type of differential diagnosis and for the complications of early pregnancy. There was a danger that we would be swamped by routine investigations and the X-ray department of the Western Infirmary have now taken on this work. I also applied the technique to the investigation of large spleens and livers and I am still seeking a reliable way of quantifying metastases in cases of hepatomegaly and should like further opportunities to distinguish the different forms of splenomegaly.

We had already noticed the very sharp echoes which were produced on either side of a baby's head and this led first of all to identifying the presentation of the fetus by finding these large echoes by just using a hand-held probe and one dimensional or A-scope presentation. My ward sister at Rottenrow, Miss Marr, now Matron of the Queen Mother's Hospital, was quick to seize on this technique in order to determine the presentation in doubtful cases in her antenatal ward before I did my grand rounds.

This led me to consider measuring the distance between the echoes as an index of the width of the head or the biparietal diameter as it is called. Experiments with metal 'heads' in water tanks showed that this was feasible and that this diameter could be very readily recognised. Mr Tom Duggan, a physicist then working with me, produced a beautiful electronic ranging unit from which the distance between echoes can be calculated directly in centimetres and millimetres. Dr Willocks, in my department, took on this subject and did many hundreds of cases with errors of less than 2 mm over 75% of cases. He further explored the rate of growth of the fetal head as an index of continuing intrauterine development.

Professor Sjovall in the University of Lund in Sweden sent one of his lecturers, Dr Sunden, to come and learn, and he eventually got a refined version of our apparatus installed in Sweden and has since reproduced our work with great thoroughness.

One of the limitations in ultrasonic diagnosis was the fact that bowel intervening between the probe and the structure one wished to examine prevented a proper investigation of organs deep in the pelvis. It occurred to me that, if we made the patient's bladder full by getting her to drink lots of tea and orange squash etc., we could transmit ultrasound through the full bladder and see the uterus or ovaries immediately behind it. This is known as the 'full bladder ultrasonogram'.

It is now possible to outline a normal uterus and we have even shown a pregnancy inside it before the urine test becomes positive. The possibility of diagnosing ectopic pregnancy, both ruptured and unruptured, is being explored.

With the commissioning of the new Queen Mother's Hospital the Department of Health for Scotland very generously offered to buy me a complete new fair copy of our original prototype apparatus and, at the time of writing, this was installed exactly one week ago and has already been put into use. This is an apparatus of immense versatility, can measure in one dimension or two, and can also display moving structures such as walls of the heart for cardiological investigation. It is quite clear that if I gave up teaching, operating and nearly all administrative and clinical work, I could spend the rest of my life fully occupied in exploring fresh fields in what is becoming a new diagnostic science. I have indeed been fortunate in the generous assistance which I have received from the firm of Smiths with the necessary engineering and electronic 'know how' and, with their factory only a few miles away across the river, I have been lucky to get a new hospital with space in which to house the equipment, and I have been lucky with my colleagues who have collaborated fully with me in what has become a very big project".

The most important paper in the early years of ultrasonic diagnosis was published in *The Lancet* of 7th June 1958. Its authors were Donald, MacVicar and Brown and the title was rather a dry one: "Investigation of abdominal masses by pulsed ultrasound". It described A-scope, B-scope and plan-position indicator (PPI) displays, discussed the apparatus, technique of scanning and results in one hundred patients.

The authors then went on to describe the possibility of harmful effects, which they reckoned were minimised by the high frequencies and low power outputs used: they considered that the harmful effects of diagnostic ultrasound were negligible. They concluded, "our findings are still of more academic interest than practical importance, and we do not feel that our clinical judgement should be influenced by our ultrasonic findings. Further refinements in technique may provide a useful diagnostic weapon in cases in which radiological diagnosis with ionising radiations is either impracticable or undesirable". These were strangely modest conclusions, coming from the principal author but, as time passed and experience increased, the confidence of the team rose.

With his forceful personality, his enthusiasm and his gift for leadership, Donald soon attracted a group of assistants who were

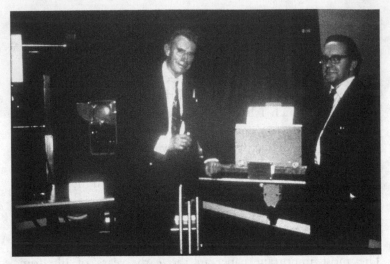

ID and T Brown inspecting old ultrasound equipment

willing to work all hours of the day to provide the technical and clinical experience that would get the project up and working.

First of these was Tom Brown. He had been working as a trainee engineer in Kelvin and Hughes and had acquired experience of design in industrial ultrasonic equipment. However, that job had been transferred elsewhere and he progressed to less exciting things. A year later he heard, quite by chance, that Professor Donald was using a flaw detector on patients and that evening he looked him up in the telephone book and made what he describes as, "the most fateful telephone call I have ever made". In a paper read to the World Ultrasound meeting in Washington in 1988 he stated "through personal contacts within the company I managed to borrow a brand new Mark IV instrument and for the next two years or so, hundreds of patients were scanned".

Brown subsequently invented a completely automatic motorised contact compound scanning machine. This went into service in 1959 and was used by Donald and his team for all the work they carried out from then until 1965.

The medical mainstay of Ian Donald's original ultrasound team at the Western Infirmary was John MacVicar. A son of the manse, from Kintyre, brought up in a very talented family, his eldest brother was Angus MacVicar, the popular novelist. Angus described their early years in two amusing autobiographical books, *Salt in my Porridge* and *Heather in my Ears*. This early upbringing smartened John up. He had a great capacity for organisation and had that down-to-earth common sense in which Ian was sometimes lacking. He did fundamental work in the study of early pregnancy and supported Ian all the way. This was not an easy task. John recollected later that the success of the original work depended on the people, the place and the time. Ian Donald was a visionary, a man of ideas, with intensive drive. As head of a university clinical department, he had access to many different patients, and these patients often worshipped the ground he walked on and therefore would allow any examination he wanted carried out. Tom Brown had the technical expertise that made him capable of acknowledging what was possible and was able to produce the machines which complemented the ideas which the clinicians gave him. John, who joined the department in 1956, described himself as "merely a young, aspiring registrar who wanted to get some work under my belt so that I would succeed in my specialist career". This is an understatement. John had ideas, intelligence and devotion to duty that showed itself in persistence where other people might have failed (he was appointed Foundation Professor in Obstetrics and Gynaecology at the University of Leicester in 1974 and set up a very successful academic and clinical department).

Acoustic coupling proved a problem initially and it was clear that Howry's waterbath technique was not applicable. John remarked, "Any of you who know Glasgow women will appreciate that it is not easy to get them into water for hygienic purposes and the idea that they would take to water for an ultra-sound examination was certainly far from the truth". Condoms and finger cots filled with water seemed a better option but they often burst, soaking the patient, the bed and the examiner!

Something else for acoustic coupling had to be found. This was olive oil, but it was messy. After a session, John and Tom Brown found their hands, cuffs, shirts, trousers, ties, handkerchief and the patients records stained with olive oil; the patient had a good wash immediately after the examination, but the examiners had some explaining to do once they got home. Despite this event, olive oil was used effectively for acoustic coupling for some time.

Ian Donald soon achieved some international recognition, particularly from the University of Lund, Sweden, which had established links with Glasgow since the time of Munro Kerr. Lund University had already produced interesting work on ultrasound, particularly the study of echo-encephalography in head injury cases by Lars Leksell, head of Lund's department of neurosurgery (1955). Leksell wrote, "The surgical results in the treatment of post-traumatic haematomata depend largely on early diagnosis, and ultrasonic examination appears promising for this purpose". Leksell had started his experiments in 1950 with a Kelvin and Hughes 'supersonic flaw detector'. Leksell's work was well known to the head of Lund's department of obstetrics and gynaecology, Professor Alf Sjövall, a gentle and genial man who stimulated research in various fields. Sjövall became friendly with Ian Donald, and in 1959 he sent Bertil Sundén, a young lecturer from his department in Lund, to Glasgow.

The consequence of his visit was that he persuaded the authorities in Lund to purchase an instrument like Donald's prototype bed-table scanner. The placing of a commercial order for such a machine (at £2,500) was a breakthrough and an enormous boost for those involved at Kelvin and Hughes. This was the very first direct-contact scanning machine to be sold commercially anywhere in the world and was the prototype of the diasonograph family of instruments. The apparatus could be used not only for two-dimensional echo recording in which a cross-sectional picture of the structures under examination was obtained but also – after changing the settings – for dimensional (A-scope) recording and for recording echoes from pulsating structures. With the aid of this machine, Sundén produced a beautifully illustrated thesis "On the diagnostic value of ultrasound in obstetrics and gynaecology" (1964). Sundén had a special interest in twins, hydramnios and fetal abnormality and produced some beautiful pictures. Ian Donald had the pleasure of going to Lund to examine Bertil Sundén on his thesis and described how the affair was conducted with full academic pomp and splendour.

In 1959, Donald noted that clear echoes could be obtained from the fetal head and began to apply this information. JW, who had joined the department in 1958, became involved in this work shortly afterwards and was given the project to play with on his own for the reason that the work had to be done where the pregnant women were, in the Royal Maternity Hospital, Rottenrow, at the other side of the city from the Western Infirmary, which the Professor had made his headquarters and which housed the compound sector scanner.

At Rottenrow, there was an old A-scan machine but there was no separate room to examine the women and not even a cupboard in which to keep the apparatus: it just stood in a corner under a sheet.

We pushed it about on a trolley and approached patients in the wards for permission to examine them at the bedside. Glasgow women are wonderful and they accepted all this without demur. A lady approached me many years later and told me that her family, whose births I had supervised, were all doing well and added "I mind ye fine, comin' roon Rottenrow wi' yer wee barra". There was, of course, no time off for research in those days and all had to be done amidst an enormous workload of emergencies in obstetrics and gynaecology, huge clinics and the teaching of undergraduates. Tom Duggan of the Western Regional Hospital Board physics department was responsible for all the technical developments and attended, often at great personal inconvenience, the examination of patients at the bedside. Work was often interrupted by clinical crises and there was one particularly dramatic day when we

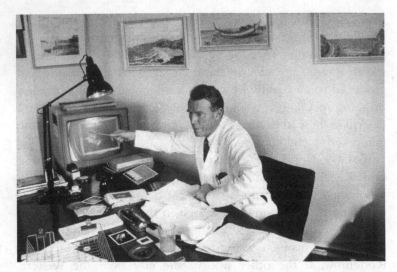

ID with TV monitor

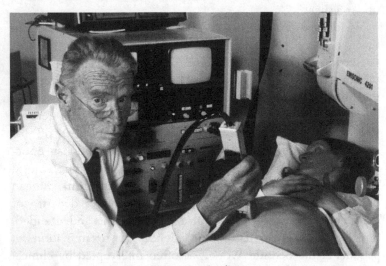

ID scanning Caroline

were trying out a new method of measurement and the whole thing had to be abandoned because the woman in the next bed started pouring blood from placenta praevia and had to be taken to theatre.

Tom Duggan perfected the technique of the electronic cursor, which produced the bright spot on the sharp echo that you obtained from the fetal head if you were examining correctly. We were then able to conduct a series of pathological studies at the same time to give some information about the speed of ultrasound in the various components of the fetal skull, scalp, bone, etc. So we were able to produce a reliable figure for converting time into distance and observing the biparietal diameter. Our use of serial measurements of the fetal head during pregnancy was the first study using ultrasound to measure fetal growth anywhere in the world.

Our results were presented at a memorable meeting of the Royal Society of Medicine in London on Friday, 12th January 1962. Professor Donald was just recovering from his first cardiac operation (a hazardous procedure in those days) and was still technically an inpatient in the Western Infirmary. MacVicar and Willocks were in attendance, somewhat apprehensive about making presentations to the august Royal Society and even more apprehensive about the state of health of the chief. It was a cold, foggy, night, not the best atmosphere for a cardiac invalid, who looked blue and breathless. The film we had prepared broke into bits on rehearsal and had to have emergency repairs. The Professor collapsed with acute dyspnoea halfway through and John MacVicar had to continue with his paper on illustrative examples of ultrasonic echograms, showing pictures of ovarian cysts, fibroids, hydatidiform mole and early pregnancy. JW then gave his paper on ultrasonic cephalometry as a measure of fetal growth in normal and abnormal pregnancy. We were all relieved when the meeting closed and breathed a great sigh of relief. In 1962, it was the first time that many people in our specialty had heard of diagnosis by ultrasound and many remained incredulous.

When the Queen Mother's Hospital opened in 1964, pregnant women had, at last, modern ultrasonic apparatus (with A- and B-scan) available to them on site. As Ian Donald said at the British Congress of Obstetrics and Gynaecology in July 1965, "The growing fetus can be repeatedly studied not only by measurement of the biparietal diameter but by fuller studies in two dimensions. The method had the advantage of subjecting the patient to neither discomfort, hazard nor indignity".

The man who became the great exponent of fetal cephalometry in two dimensions – a technique which had not been available before – was Stuart Campbell. He came to a junior post in the Queen Mother's Hospital in 1965 and worked initially with James Willocks, whom he described as "the man with the machine". He has vivid recollections of Ian Donald "who was really quite an intimidating senior doctor. He always asked quick unexpected questions – and did have a quick temper. I just learned to be quiet and he soon calmed down, because he was an extraordinarily generous man". Stuart Campbell moved to London in 1968, taking up a post as lecturer in Queen Charlotte's Maternity Hospital under Professor Sir John Dewhurst, who encouraged him greatly. He became Professor of Obstetrics and Gynaecology at King's College Hospital in 1976, moving to St George's Hospital in 1996. Throughout his career he has done much to publicise ultrasound and has become an international celebrity.

Another arrival in Glasgow in 1965 was Usama Abdulla from Baghdad. Ian Donald had visited Iraq as a guest of Professor Kamal Samarrae, who was Usama's chief. Ian said to Usama, "Would you like to come and learn about a new technique which I have developed called ultrasound?". Professor Samarrae, attended by Abdulla, came to the British Congress in Glasgow in 1965 and Usama stayed on. His great work with Professor Donald was on placentography (1968). This was of fundamental importance clinically, for placenta praevia is a potentially dangerous and life-threatening condition because of haemorrhage. If the position of the placenta is shown clearly, appropriate action can be taken. Usama moved to Queen Charlotte's in London, then eventually to Oxford and Liverpool Universities, where he helped to establish the first ultrasound department in each of these cities.

The next important arrival was Hugh Robinson, who arrived as a research registrar in 1971, becoming lecturer from 1976 to 1978, when he moved to the Department of Obstetrics and Gynaecology, University of Melbourne, Australia. When Hugh came to the Queen Mother's Hospital he was looking for a research project and JW suggested to him that he could use ultrasound in the assessment of women with threatened and incomplete miscarriage, who took up a lot of space in the gynaecology department of the Western Infirmary. This went on to a wide-ranging study of problems in early pregnancy and eventually to the early display of fetal heart activity (1972). Hugh Robinson reported that the presence or absence of fetal heart movement might be reliably detected by an abdominal approach from the forty-eighth day of pregnancy onwards (menstrual age). This was a discovery of fundamental clinical importance and it made clinical management much easier.

In a conversation in October 2002, Hugh recalled Ian Donald with great affection. When he submitted some important work to him, the Professor remarked wearily "O, Hugh, I wish you wouldn't split infinitives!". Hugh said that he did not even know what a split infinitive was, but he welcomed the help. Ian Donald supported everything that Hugh did. He found the Professor's approach broadminded. It was as if he opened a gate to a new field and said, "Go in. Cultivate it as you like!". Hugh Robinson believed that Ian Donald had his own vision of his ultrasonic world, but it was not a concept cast in stone. His most telling observations were anecdotal, relating to patients that he knew, and evidence-based medicine was not really his scene; but, as has been said, he was never dull.

Ultrasound barely avoided a severe crash in 1966 when the Kelvin and Hughes Glasgow factory, now part of Smith's Industrial Division, was closed. Professor Donald wrote,

"Desperately I could see our apparatus suffering the fate of so much electronic apparatus in medicine – namely the dustsheet phenomenon". Again, he approached the University Principal, now Sir Charles Wilson, who instructed him to set up his own department and to engage John Fleming and Angus Hall, members of the original team, as research engineers.

Following their valuable experience working on medical ultrasound projects in these firms, their talents were a great asset. John Fleming had a special working relationship with Hugh Robinson, establishing the measurement of fetal crown–rump length, which is still in use today. John Fleming was also aware that there was a lot of ultrasonic apparatus that was of great historical interest. Without some intervention it was likely to be thrown on the rubbish dump. He saved it and is now coordinator of the British Medical Ultrasound Society (BMUS) collection and keeper of ultrasonic equipment in the Hunterian Museum, University of Glasgow. Angus Hall trained as a Merchant Navy radio officer before joining Kelvin and Hughes in 1957 and working on medical ultrasonic diagnosis. He was President of BMUS in 1981–82 and since 1982 has been Head of Medical Physics at St James' University Hospital, Leeds. He was Chairman of the Wellcome Trust Seminar, "Looking at the unborn", which is such a valuable source of recollections. Without Fleming and Hall, who understood the subject so well, development would have been less smooth and less successful. After Angus Hall's appointment to Leeds, John Fleming remained in Glasgow, providing ingenuity, ideas and endless patience to the development of ultrasound.

A third important member of the team was, and is, Jonathan Powell, technician and mechanical wizard: "Jack of all trades and master of some", as he describes himself. His previous passions for motor cars, clocks and radios have all proved invaluable in the developments in ultrasonic research. To walk into his laboratory is like entering a scene that only Heath Robinson could have drawn and yet among it all is science and clarity.

Despite his poor health since 1961, the sixties were a time of great success for Ian Donald. He acquired much international fame, particularly in the USA, where he had excellent relationships with Louis Hellman of New York and Joseph Holmes of Denver. Horace Thompson, at the University of Colorado, had been in the ultrasound business since the time of Douglass Howry's work in the early 1950s. Horace Thompson said about Ian Donald, "We were in touch from the time I started. I visited with him, he visited with us, we compared notes. Yes, there was competition, but it was a friendly competition because there were never any harsh feelings about what we were doing".

An American Gynaecological Visiting Society was invited to Glasgow in May 1968 and the members were lyrical about what they saw and the friendly reception they were given.

As a result of his American contacts, Ian Donald was invited to give the prestigious Joseph Price Oration, presented at the 79th Annual Meeting of the American Association of Obstetricians and Gynecologists in Hot Springs, Virginia, 5th to 7th September 1968. Ian had now cast aside any diffidence he had possessed about the subject of ultrasound and entitled his lecture "On launching a new diagnostic science", a high-sounding title. He pointed out that it would not be the first time in history that obstetrics and gynaecology had provided a growing point towards a wider horizon in scientific thinking, instancing Simpson in anaesthesia, Semmelweis in the fight against puerperal sepsis, and pioneers of abdominal surgery like Robert Houston and Ephraim McDowell, the first to operate safely on ovarian cysts.

In the twentieth century, the first effective use of sulphonamides was in puerperal sepsis and the first effective radiotherapy was in treatment of cancer of the cervix. "Is it too much to claim, I wonder, that history may be in the process of repeating itself?" He went on to contrast the history of medical ultrasound and radiology. "There are some striking contrasts. For one thing, radiology owes its origins practically entirely to one man, whose name has been given to the subject as a whole. William Conrad Roentgen first became interested in cathode rays at 50 years of age and in November 1958 discovered X-rays. Three quite brief publications in the course of the next eighteen months, two of them in the none too widely read *Proceedings of the Würzburg Physical Medical Society*, were sufficient to excite the interest of the entire civilised world and, within a few months, the discovery of X-rays became front page news in England where the Roentgen Society was formed in 1897. There followed a period of intense amateurish activity when radiologists were also their own physicists and technicians and it was a couple of decades before reasonably reliable equipment became commercially available. In sonar, on the other hand, we seem to have crept in behind the maternal skirts of modern engineering, availing ourselves of the cast-offs and behaving, at least until recently, very much like poor cousins. Yet it is possible that the dazzling start of the first half-century of radiology may yet be overtaken by the more steady and highly controlled growth of ultrasonic diagnosis. Sonar must, however, in no sense be regarded as an alternative to standard radiology but rather as an adjuvant technique which I feel must ultimately be embraced by the world of radiology at large."

It is interesting to note that Lord Kelvin, founder of the Kelvin and Hughes Company, Professor of Natural Philosophy at the University of Glasgow, five times President of the Royal Society and a giant of Victorian science, had a contact with Roentgen. When Roentgen made his sensational discovery of X-rays he hastened to inform Kelvin, who received his letter in December 1895 at about the same time as Roentgen's first publication. Kelvin was "astonished and delighted" and thanked Roentgen for "so early sending me your paper and the photographs". However, Kelvin, aged seventy-one, was in bed with a blood clot in the leg and pleurisy so was unable to pursue the matter personally. He passed the information on to his nephew and assistant, the physicist Dr JT Bottomley, who in turn passed it to Dr John McIntyre, who founded, in Glasgow Royal Infirmary, the first department of clinical radiology in the United Kingdom and probably in the world.

To return to Ian's Joseph Price Oration, he continued:

"It will be appreciated that ultrasonic energy has a completely different spectrum of activity from that of electromagnetic energy which includes light, heat and X-rays, and other forms of ionising radiation, and therefore ultrasound provides a very different type of information yield from shadow pictures resulting from X-rays. Because different tissues transmit and reflect ultrasound differently according to their physical properties, soft tissue studies become possible, and here we should not forget the original pioneer work in the United States by Wild, Howry, Reid and Bliss in the early 1950s.

We ourselves were relatively latecomers, only entering the field in 1955. Wild, for example, sought to measure the thickness of bowel wall and hence signs of carcinomatous ulceration of the stomach using a quartz transducer within the lumen of the gut. His experiments were carried out on dead dogs' intestines and postmortem-room material. Having never had to waste time myself on animals and corpses, both of which I detest in experimental work, I was able to cut a lot of the corners which they had first to round. The use of high-frequency ultrasonic waves for detecting changes in the texture of living tissues led to the hope that hitherto undiagnosed malignancy within the breast might be thereby revealed; but with wavelengths measurable in sizeable fractions of a millimetre it would indeed be asking a lot of a new technique such as this to rival the refinement of proper histological diagnosis, and no surgeon would rest content with anything less. This kind of digression serves to remind one that the tool should fit the problem, rather than the problem made to fit the available tool. More sophisticated techniques were soon developed by the Denver team, whose members I regard proudly as rivals and friends.

The echo information supplied by a single scanning beam is difficult to unravel unless it is depicted in two dimensions at least, and Howry and Bliss produced, I believe, the first two-dimensional sonograms in 1950. Again, their work unfortunately was confined largely to postmortem room material, although they noted that better pictures could be obtained from the fresh specimens of living subjects than formalin-fixed specimens. We soon found this out ourselves and threw our tanks on to the top of the most inaccessible cupboards. As soon as we got rid of the backroom attitude and brought our apparatus fully into the department with an inexhaustible supply of living patients with fascinating clinical problems we were able to get ahead really fast.

Clinical usefulness of sonar[1]

Any new knowledge or technique becomes more attractive if its clinical usefulness can be demonstrated without harm, indignity, or discomfort to the patient; better still if it requires not the eye of faith to comprehend it, or as Shakespeare said in a different context, in King Lear, "Get thee glass eyes and, like a scurvy politician, seem to see the things thou dost not". Comprehension as I shall briefly show you is well within the range of any average clinician. Our turnover is now very large and running usually at over 200 cases a month. In fact in the midst of exploring new territory we are having to provide a diagnostic service, often from far afield. The setting up of two more ultrasonic units within the City of Glasgow has tended to increase our workload by popularising the technique rather than to diminish it, as originally intended, and the demand in snowballing.

At present, the most widely used clinical application of sonar is in the diagnosis of head injuries where the

---

1 Sonar' was Ian Donald's preferred term for diagnostic ultrasound. It eventually was displaced by the simple word 'ultrasound'.

detection of midline shifts caused by extradural bleeding may help to distinguish the case from one of alcoholic stupor or some other cause of unconsciousness. This is a simple application involving the use of A-scan where the echoes are represented as vertical blips and whose depth corresponds to their distance toward the right along a time-based sweep on a cathode ray tube. The other principal use for unidimensional A-scan work is in the measurement of the fetal biparietal diameter, which has now come to be widely exploited. It is when we come to pregnancy and its complications that we meet the richest strike of all. There is not so much difference after all between a fetus in utero and a submarine at sea.

It is simply a question of refinement. Also, placentography by sonar has now become such standard practice in our part of the world that it has displaced all other methods.

Safety of sonar

Since ultrasound is a form of mechanical energy it would be reasonable to expect that at some threshold level trauma could be inflicted and that different tissues would have different susceptibilities. High-power concentrated ultrasonic energy has indeed been known to be damaging, and nervous tissue is reputed to be more susceptible than other structures. At the very-low-power outputs employed in sonar as distinct from industrial and therapeutic applications there is extraordinarily little evidence so far of damaging effect; in fact none at all.

To us as obstetricians the possibly damaging effects upon early embryonic life are particularly important and the utmost vigilance must be maintained because in the future more sophisticated and more powerful machines may one day introduce a hazard at present hardly foreseen, let alone understood. We must not forget that it took nearly half a century for the damaging effects of X-rays upon the fetus *in utero* to come to light. Alas we hardly yet know in which direction to look.

Making a start

In medicine today there are two main types of research, the animate and the inanimate. Inanimate research usually involves the measurement of some property, be it trace element, enzyme or structural feature on a portable specimen removed far from the scene of the patient's illness. Such specimens may include blood, serum, urine, faeces and a variety of expendable tissues. While not denying its importance, there are many of us for whom such activities hold very little attraction and we prefer a more animated type of research, on the patient, with the patient, as far as possible by the patient and, always, for the patient. To produce a technical trick with apparatus, however ingenious, is not enough. The clinical work to which you and I are dedicated demands something of demonstrable clinical value and this is where gynaecology above all wins.

Anyone who is satisfied with his diagnostic ability and with his surgical results is unlikely to contribute much to the launching of a new medical science. He should first be consumed with a divine discontent with things as they are. It greatly helps, of course, to have the right idea at the right time, and quite good ideas may come, Archimedes fashion, in one's bath. This, however, is the easiest part of all and the real tussle comes with trying to put the idea into practice. The inevitable disappointment that usually appears early on may strangle the idea at its very birth. There is need, therefore, for a combination of enthusiasm and sufficient ignorance to prevent the loss of momentum before getting truly under way. Very high on the list of prerequisites for a successful launching is the phenomenon of 'beginner's luck', of which I have had more than my share even allowing for the statement by Louis Pasteur that, "In observation luck only follows minds prepared for it". In other words, the chance observation and the prepared mind. The mind, however, can only be prepared by being already committed to the project. There is, however, danger in the preconceived notion because it may easily develop into an intellectual blind spot and Claude Bernard, that famous Parisian physiologist, reminded the world that it is what we think we know that prevents us from learning. On the other hand, erudite caution can be a handicap too, forcing the conclusion upon the indolent that the whole problem is too difficult to tackle, and in the words of Hamlet:

> "Thus the native hue of resolution
> Is sicklied o'er with the pale cast of thought,
> And enterprises of great pith and moment
> With this regard their currents turn awry
> And lose the name of action."

All experimentation must leave room for failure, since failure is far more instructive than success. To fail and to start again is like embarking upon a second marriage which Dr Samuel Johnson, the famous English lexicographer, described as a "triumph of hope over experience".

Attitude of colleagues

In medicine learning is indivisible. I have always regretted the appearance of any segregation between the so-called "pure" clinician and the not so pure academic type, and likewise I have always deplored the talk about the art of obstetrics as though it were something more lofty than obstetric science. Fortunately, this attitude does not seriously prevail in the United States and certainly not in

Scotland, where to misquote Shakespeare who was really talking about Kings, "There is such divinity doth hedge a professor that treason can but peep to what it would". In England the academic worker has all too often been regarded as a lower form of less inspired life.

The attitude of colleagues can make or mar a new project. In the same way that a housewife is reputed to get the servants she deserves, an investigator usually gets the colleagues he deserves too. It would be a pleasant form of self-flattery to enlarge upon this theme, but it must suffice to acknowledge my indebtedness to my own colleagues. The danger arises when the credulity of colleagues becomes uncritical. Happy indeed is the man who like myself has colleagues who both understand the scope of sonar and know its limitations, and this diagnostic service now runs as well whether I am at home or abroad – surely the hallmark of a good department.

I have given a brief account of the past, an outline of present usage, and would now like to take a cautious look into the future. One thing is certain – those of us already in this field will not do worse but only better than has already been done.

Conclusion

Mr President, I put it to you and to the members of this Association that the case for sonar as a diagnostic tool has been made out amply by its demonstrated usefulness in obstetrics and gynaecology. Can any major diagnostic unit in the civilised world within the next fifteen years afford to do without a diagnostic aid so basically simple and direct? The radiologist of tomorrow who persists in ignoring what sonar has to offer will be like the cardiologist of yesterday who spurned electrocardiography.

I will therefore end by quoting from Lewis Carroll's *Alice in Wonderland*:

> "Will you walk a little faster
> Said the whiting to the snail
> There's a porpoise just behind me
> And he's treading on my tail
> See how eagerly the lobsters
> And the turtles all advance
> They are awaiting on the shingle
> Won't you come and join the dance?"

The Joseph Price oration was in truth a bravura performance. To us it is the most vivid, stimulating and amusing of all the many lectures he gave on the development of ultrasound as his fame increased. And increase it certainly did.

At home, Dr Ellis Barnett, consultant radiologist, became fascinated with medical ultrasound when he worked at the Glasgow Royal Maternity Hospital. Later, with the introduction of medical ultrasound to the radiology department at the Western Infirmary, Ellis Barnett made an enormous contribution, training many overseas radiologists and publishing many papers. The textbook *Clinical Diagnostic Ultrasound*, by Drs Barnett and Patricia Morley, was for many years a leading authority in the field and attracted many international visitors to the Western Infirmary. Barnett and Morley were not confined to gynaecological diagnosis and awoke their clinical colleagues to the possibilities of this "new diagnostic science" in cardiology, renal medicine and surgery and other branches.

In Bristol, Professor Peter Wells, medical physicist, began work on medical ultrasound in 1960 and from 1963 was concerned with developments in diagnostic methods. He became a firm friend of Tom Brown, Angus Hall and John Fleming. This relationship was productive on both sides. Later, in 1998, Peter Wells was awarded the Ian Donald Medal for Technical Merit by the International Society of Ultrasound in Obstetrics and Gynaecology.

Dr Tony Whittingham, physicist, taught ultrasound, beginning in Aberdeen and later becoming Head of the Ultrasonics section at the Medical Physics Department at Newcastle General Hospital. He pioneered the development of linear-array in the UK and later helped in persuading Glasgow University to look after the historical collection of ultrasound equipment made by John Fleming. These are just a few examples of the interest stimulated by ultrasound in Britain.

On the clinical side, it is noteworthy that Stuart Campbell, with his enthusiasm, converted many London obstetricians and gynaecologists to the value of diagnostic ultrasound – a hard job.

In Europe, a noteworthy figure was Alfred Kratochwil of Vienna, who was an obstetrician. After Kratochwil learned of Donald, MacVicar and Brown's work, he persuaded the Kretz Company to develop a B-scanner. This instrument facilitated additional clinical applications, which enabled Kratochwil to make a major contribution to the development of ultrasonic imaging. Initial scepticism from his colleagues was replaced by enormous enthusiasm and interdisciplinary cooperation, which led to foundation of a European ultrasound diagnostic and training centre in October 1970, small enough that doctors of all medical specialties met daily and were well informed: an atmosphere similar to that of the Queen Mother's Hospital.

In Australia, the ultrasonic pioneers George Kossoff and Bill Garrett were concerned by a report by Dr Alice Stewart (1956) suggesting a link between childhood leukaemia and X-ray examination in pregnancy and experimented with ultrasound images of the pregnant uterus (1962). Their first international publication was in 1966 and they introduced grey-scale imaging in 1969.

Reference has already been made to Ian Donald's close relationship with American colleagues, particularly in Denver, Colorado but he made many overseas tours in the 1960s. In 1968, he returned to the country of his youth, South Africa, as a guest lecturer and, needless to say, his topic was "The use and application of diagnostic ultrasound".

Among the audience were Professors Dennis Davey and Leon Van Dongen (we knew Leon Van Dongen had Glasgow connections by marriage, but we never met him). Leon Van Dongen's request was turned down as "a newfangled gimmick" (he was later successful). Davey was successful in his request for support and this was the beginning of ultrasound in South Africa.

Two years later an article was produced suggesting that chromosome damage was caused by ultrasound (Macintosh and Davey, 1970). The research was repeated in other centres without damage being found but Davey's association with the report hurt Ian Donald deeply, as he was a former pupil of Ian's in London. It was five years later before the authors of the damaging report withdrew their allegations.

The spread of ultrasound in obstetrics remained unchecked and numerous new techniques were applied, details of which can be found in the superb review by Margaret McNay and John Fleming "Forty years of obstetric ultrasound 1957–1997; from A-scope to three dimensions".

When Ian Donald retired in 1976, his successor, Professor Charles Whitfield, continued to support new work on ultrasound. Dr Margaret McNay developed the clinical application of ultrasound from 1978 to 1996 in the Queen Mother's Hospital, where she was consultant and head of the department of obstetric ultrasound. Her main interest was in the prenatal diagnosis of congenital abnormalities and fetal therapy.

In the fetal therapy field, her colleagues were Martin Whittle and David Gilmore (who died in his forties in 2002). Martin Whittle was 'talent-spotted' by Professor Charles Whitfield in his Manchester days and was persuaded to come to Glasgow. He was later appointed as Professor of Fetal Medicine at Birmingham.

Ultrasound has continued to attract young doctors – the thrill of seeing the baby in the womb cannot be equalled, just as the birth of a baby remains a thrill to the obstetrician until retirement. But increasing precision can bring its problems. Some of these were identified by Professor Martin Whittle in his Ian

Donald Memorial Lecture, delivered in Glasgow in November 2002, at a commemorative meeting for David Gilmore. He entitled it "Light from sound" and in it he gave a detailed account of antenatal screening. Some of his conclusions were:

- Ultrasound has transformed obstetric management.
- Its value as a screening test for fetal abnormalities remains uncertain: harm versus benefit must be assessed.
- Ultrasonographers must be clear of the purpose of the scan before its performance.
- Ultrasound scanning for fetal abnormalities should be to an agreed set of standards.
- Where these standards cannot be met the continuing use of ultrasound should be reconsidered.

These conclusions are based on a vast experience of fetal medicine and Ian Donald would have approved, for he was always afraid that the popularity of ultrasound scanning could have its dark side.

Another fetal medicine specialist is Kypros Nicolaides, who conveys some of the thrill of the work. He studied medicine at King's College in London. As a fourth-year medical student he was a pupil of Stuart Campbell. Kypros records, "After seeing moving images I fell in love with that area of medicine. I just wanted to become a fetal medicine doctor. Here was the whole of postnatal medicine to a new patient who has now become visible, therefore accessible. If babies are anaemic, you find out why they are anaemic and treat them". Kypros Nicolaides became a Professor in 1992 and in 1996 he established the Fetal Medicine Foundation, which runs regular courses. He continues to be fascinated by fetal medicine applying the principles and techniques of postnatal medicine to prenatal life. Considering the ethical implications is a constant challenge. "The combination of these" says Kypros, "keeps you on your toes. There's a lot of excitement, a lot of sadness, a lot of depression, but a lot of emotion. So it never becomes boring". A great many people come to him expecting miracles. So how does he cope?

He says, "I never sit down and wonder how I cope. I just get into it. It's not a job. It's my life!".

Kypros was recently awarded the Ian Donald Gold Medal for the highest contribution in ultrasound from the International Society of Ultrasound in Obstetrics and Gynaecology. Ian Donald would have been proud of him. He displays that spirit, that "smeddum" which Ian always admired.

Ian Donald's legacy is alive and well with supporters like these.

Home Life and Hobbies

In 1937, Ian married Alix Mathide Richards, daughter of a farmer in the Orange Free State. Happily married for fifty years he was the loving father of four daughters. We met Alix and the family last at the naming of the Ian Donald Fetal Medicine Unit in the Queen Mother's Hospital on 1st July, 2003.

Each of his four daughters, born at seven-year intervals, displayed characteristics of their father. Tessa is a commanding figure, a Norwegian citizen, who has given up a successful career in medicine and taken up painting, one of her father's hobbies. Christina lives in the Orkney Islands managing a croft, taking time out to play the oboe professionally and to teach wind instruments. She features annually in the St. Magnus Festival in Kirkwall. Caroline stays in Deal not far from her mother and is a cellist. Her husband makes and repairs stringed instruments. Margaret ("Noggy") is a record-breaker. She got married at seventeen years of age (her mother was eighteen) and lives happily with her family.

The family home was a grey sandstone villa in the west end of Glasgow occupied by Ian, Alix and their four daughters. Alix was wonderful. Half South African, half French, she was the perfect foil for Ian and was able to provide a calm, if occasionally slightly disordered, background for his constantly active and restless way of life. She is one of the few women we know who could remain unperturbed by the announcement from Ian late in the afternoon that he was bringing home three guests for supper and would then conjure up a delightful meal over which she would preside with complete equanimity.

Ian's hobbies were sailing, painting and enjoyment of classical music. He had no interest whatsoever in sport. Having been schooled in Fettes, he could just about differentiate a rugby ball from a soccer ball and he would not have known a Rangers or Celtic jersey if it appeared in his front garden. When asked if he played golf he always replied by saying "When I became a man I put away childish things" and always described golf clubs as golf sticks.

He was equally disinterested in gardening and could not or would not differentiate one plant or flower or shrub from another. Fortunately, they had only a small garden, which Alix did her best to keep in order.

His interest and love for sailing were stimulated during holidays from school which he spent with a cousin from Paisley, Archie Craig, whose family had a holiday house in the Kyles of Bute. They also had a sailing boat in which the boys spent many happy days exploring the Firth of Clyde.

Ian's first boat in Glasgow was a Daily Mirror dinghy constructed from a kit. It was kept in the front hall of the house and had to be circumnavigated by all visitors on entering. At weekends, the boat was trailed behind the family Dormobile to Helensburgh, where it was put in the water. He was an expert sailor and, as a natural teacher, was delighted when I (WB) asked him to instruct me in the rudiments of the sport.

On these occasions we were sometimes accompanied by Jacques, the family dog, a white French poodle. I well recollect the occasion when we stopped in Dumbarton to allow Jacques to relieve himself. So engrossed did Ian become in the intricacies of handling a boat that we quite forgot about Jacques and proceeded on our way. Half an hour later we noticed his absence and there followed a turnabout and a frenzied search of the streets until we finally located him. Ian was much relieved as Jacques was really Alix's dog and to have returned without him would have made him less than popular.

The second boat was much larger (about twenty feet) and was built in his garage with his own hands from the bare wood which he bought and fashioned lovingly into the curved planks which constitute the clinker type of construction seen in the traditional herring boats plying the waters of the Clyde estuary

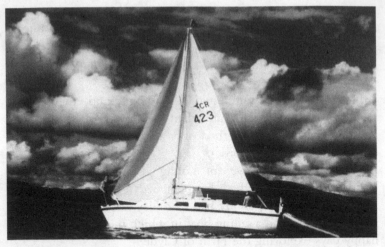
Sailing on Loch Fyne

but, alas, gradually disappearing as fish stocks lessen and foreign competition increases despite attempts to regulate the size and number of catches.

I (WB) was roped in to assist with the building of this boat when an extra pair of hands was needed, and I well remember the laying of the keel. It was fashioned from an enormous length of mahogany and Ian decided to shape it by the traditional method of using an adze. This was a terrifying procedure, an adze consisting of a razor sharp curved blade attached to a handle and manipulated by swinging it horizontally between one's feet. A misdirected blow would almost certainly result in serious injury or even amputation of his foot and I was much relieved when that part of the boat's construction was completed without serious mishap.

By the time it was completed he had acquired the extended use of a cottage on the shores of Loch Fyne, loaned to him by Lady Lindsay, an ex-patient who owned an estate in that part of the country. This was ideal for the family and many happy weekends were spent in these waters, which were ideal for his type of sailing.

When at sea and within sight of the cottage he had an elaborate system of communication for the occasions when he had to keep in touch with the hospital. He would keep his eye on the cottage and, if he was wanted, a red blanket would be waved frantically from an upstairs window and then a small dinghy would row him ashore. On one such occasion Drs Wishart and Crawford, whose sardonic wit has already been reported, were heard to remark "He didn't need the dinghy – he could have walked on the water".

Jonathan Powell, the multitalented technician in the Queen Mother's Hospital Laboratory, tells an amusing story about a trip to Loch Fyne. Early in the morning, the Professor came to him and announced, "I have declared today a departmental holiday and think we should take a trip to the seaside". The ulterior motive was soon apparent. The engine in his boat at Loch Fyne was not working well and he wanted Jonathan to mend it. Jonathan got some essential tools ready and Ian, Alix and he set off. When they arrived Ian said, "Where is the battery, sweetheart?". Alix replied, "I do not have it darling, you have it". When the truth dawned that no battery was with them, they set off again on the long return drive to Glasgow. Ian thought the best thing was to go back to the Queen Mother's Hospital and consult his secretary Adèle Ure. When he got there, he stormed in, saying "Where is the battery for my boat?". Adèle, always imperturbable, said quietly, "Where you left it – in my office". So the three of them, with battery, returned to Loch Fyne, the battery was fitted, the engine mended and a chastened absent-minded Professor returned home.

His other hobbies were painting and music. His paintings were mostly in oil and were of landscapes in various parts of Scotland. They were formal in character and pleasant to the eye.

His love of music was inherited from his mother who had been a concert pianist and at every available opportunity he could be found at the piano playing from the music of his beloved Beethoven or Chopin. It was a sense of regret to him that all his other activities left little time for practice.

"Naught for your comfort"

Social change and medical controversy

"Naught for your comfort" is a quotation from G K Chesterton's *Ballad of the White Horse* and was used by Ian Donald as the title for his Charter Day Lecture at the National Maternity Hospital, Dublin on 10th June 1972. In it, he discussed medical ethics in our specialty. "Something momentous is happening right now in our subject of obstetrics and gynaecology. In fact, ethical issues crop up more in the gynaecologist's practice today than in any other branch of medicine." The 1960s and 70s were certainly a momentous era and to understand the problems we must cast our minds back from the twenty-first century, with its acceptance of 'patient power'.

The modern point of view was well expressed by Melanie Reid, in *The Herald*, 9th July, 2002, a newspaper columnist writing about some hostile comments that had been made about the increased availability of the 'abortion pill'. She wrote, "Developments which improve the quality of women's lives are invariably criticised for being too easy: anything which gives women less work, more time, and better control of their own bodies is greeted with suspicion and resentment. Many of the most fervent anti-abortionists are men, motivated by an apparent desire to control women's bodies, and utterly incapable of understanding the desperation of a woman facing an unwanted child. We live in an increasing sexualised society, where more and more people are consumers. Like it or not, sex is now deregulated and is regarded as a mainstream leisure activity. You don't need a licence, a driving test or any exam passes. This is the way things are, and we need to get real. We can never turn back the clock to stop intervention in the life cycle. It would be unfair because a woman, as an individual, has the right to choose what to do with her own body, and the right to have that decision acted on as swiftly and sensibly as possible. The current row over medical abortion is wholly phoney, whipped up by people who claim to be compassionate about unborn life, but do so at the expense of the suffering of the living. The fuss will die down and the abortion pill will continue to save women's lives and mental health".

This is a clear exposition of the current liberal feminist point of view. As such, it is politically correct.

It certainly needs a leap of the imagination to take us back to the 1960s, when the arguments that meant so much to Ian Donald were taking place. The whole debate was extremely important in his life from then on. The Kinsey report on sexual behaviour had been published in 1948 and the contraceptive pill was introduced in 1952, but it was in the sixties that their impact was really felt. As the poet Philip Larkin wrote, nostalgically:

"Sexual intercourse began in nineteen sixty-three
It was rather late for me".

Contraception was, of course, the most important influence. The disciples of Marie Stopes rejoiced. Eminent medical men were also involved in the trend towards *liberalis*. A landmark case was that of Alec Bourne, the London gynaecologist who was prosecuted for performing an abortion. It is described in more detail below.

The greatest and most influential voice in favour of liberalising abortion was that of Scotland's most eminent obstetrician and gynaecologist, Sir Dugald Baird. He delivered the Sandoz Lecture which he entitled "The Fifth Freedom" on the problems of world population and unwanted pregnancy, which was published in the British Medical Journal of 13th November 1965. Churchill and Roosevelt, during the Second World War had proclaimed "Four Freedoms" as their aim –

freedom of speech, freedom of religion, freedom from want and freedom from fear. To these Baird added a "Fifth Freedom" – freedom from the tyranny of excessive fertility.

Practising in Glasgow in the 1930s, Baird was appalled at the conditions in which women had their confinements at home. He was also shocked by the high maternal and infant mortality rates in the Glasgow Royal Maternity Hospital, where two mothers died each week from complications of childbirth. He realised the importance of social factors in obstetrics. When he moved to Aberdeen in 1937, he introduced epidemiology into obstetric practice and was the founder of social obstetrics. He created the first free family planning clinic in Britain, offered abortion to Aberdeen women and encouraged women who had completed their family to be sterilised.

The lecture of the "Fifth Freedom" was sincere, rational and well organised, reflecting his professional practice. His philosophy and practice was keenly disputed by Ian Donald. On 22nd November 1965, Ian sent a letter off to the *BMJ* in response to Sir Dugald's lecture. We, his colleagues, subscribed to it after making some emendations by removing a few inflammatory sentences (Ian was always a "bonny fechter" and sometimes went over the top in expressing his views).

We reproduce the letter here because it states clearly and eloquently what Ian thought about this important issue, which was to influence him throughout the rest of his life. We reproduce it also because it remained unpublished.

"The Editor
British Medical Journal
BMA House
Tavistock Square
LONDON WC1

Sir,

Freedom to Destroy Life

Sir Dugald Baird in his Sandoz Lecture (published in the *British Medical Journal* of the 13th November 1965) has surveyed the problem of world over-population, (which means other people's children) and has attempted to link it with the more individual problem of the unwanted pregnancy, which is a very different matter. It is in acknowledgement of Sir Dugald's great authority and unquestioned sincerity that we feel collectively bound to state our opposition to some at least of his well-intentioned, but nevertheless dangerous arguments.

Only better education and rising social conditions will bring about a greater sense of responsibility in parenthood. Therapeutic abortion will not increase it nor do anything to solve the circumstances which have made pregnancy unwelcome. The case for sterilisation is more easily made out but the performance of a practically irreversible operation such as tubal ligation in young multiparous women, who might become widows, remarry and wish to rear a second family, in spite of their present attitudes, seems unnecessarily drastic when modern contraceptive techniques are increasingly available. There is a big difference, however, between the prevention of conception and the destruction of a life already conceived.

In considering termination of pregnancy we must first of all distinguish clearly between cases in which prolongation of pregnancy is, in itself, dangerous by delaying life-saving treatment which might be incompatible with fetal survival, (for example, cases of carcinoma of the cervix in pregnancy) and on the other hand where it is simply a case of a baby unwanted because of inconvenience, expense or nuisance value, the prospect of which is undermining maternal morale and psychological health. It is seldom pregnancy per se which endangers the mother's life or health, even her mental health, in these days of modern antenatal care and hospital facilities, but it is usually the unfortunate baby, or the thought of it, that may drive a woman to desperation and doctors to a sympathetic desire to help her. Baird has gone to great lengths to seek expert advice in assessing social and psychiatric problems but his work may influence others less objectively critical to extend the indications for abortion to a degree he would not endorse. Decisions become more painful when there is reason to suspect the normality of the fetus. To burden a family and society with a seriously handicapped child makes one pause to think but society does not tolerate the liquidation, for example, of hydrocephalic babies that survive birth and modern paediatric surgeons go to great lengths to save what they can. Yet the possibility and not even the certainty of a handicapped child, for example following rubella in early pregnancy, is accepted by some as a valid indication to terminate the pregnancy. Baird's cases, however, do not apparently consist of these not very common tragedies, but deal with such matters as multiparity and "debility", social conditions and psychiatric instability. Debility is an imprecise diagnosis from a centre renowned for its accuracy in scientific thinking.

Anaemia and malnutrition are treatable, pregnant or not, and poverty can be mitigated by intelligently run social services in which Aberdeen is pre-eminent.

The law, as it stands, evidently needs no relaxation when one observes the impunity with which Baird has exercised his privilege as a doctor to end pregnancies because of his sincere opinion that such action was in the patient's interests.

Much can be done, short of termination, to help parents faced with an unintentional and therefore unwanted pregnancy and it is clear that Sir Dugald has had considerable success in this respect for which many patients, and certainly their once threatened surviving offspring have cause to be grateful. But the cases in which he has failed and where he has resorted to the expedient of termination are disturbing. It is well recognised that many marriages turn out to be sordid and unhappy but there are less disagreeable and more effective methods of dealing with the problem than obliterating the unwelcome pregnancies that result from them. Many parents faced with an unplanned pregnancy would at some time or other welcome riddance of it but they come to terms with it and soon the new baby becomes an important member of the family circle. To remind them at this stage of their previous intent would horrify them.

Therapeutic abortion in two percent of all maternities in Aberdeen is indeed a striking figure and if applied to the whole country would mean more than 17,000 terminations a year. It has to be fairly admitted that the incidence of criminal abortion in other cities, like our own, is probably many times higher. Baird suggests that in Aberdeen the unqualified criminal abortionist does not flourish and thinks that this may be due to the attitude of the local members of the medical profession. It is, of course, possible that canny Aberdonians did not offer much of a living to the abortionist even before the days of Baird's own influence on his colleagues.

He gives no comparative statistics. Our own gynae-cological unit has its full share of leftover work from the ministrations of these individuals and thanks to modern therapy the patients make good recoveries. We disagree that it is our function to become the abortionists.

Sometimes the suggestion to terminate a pregnancy because of a possible medical hazard comes first, not from the patient herself, but from her doctor. We feel that such an opinion should not be voiced to the patient until the decision is made by the gynaecologist with whom the ultimate responsibility must always lie. Fortunately this is a rare occurrence in our area, depressed though it may be, and reflects the prevailing medical philosophy for which the teaching hospitals are largely responsible. If pressures operate differently in the north east of Scotland it is perhaps because of a different philosophy in the medical school. We feel bound to assert a contrary point of view, hence the purpose of this letter which while fully appreciating the Aberdonian efforts to face a big problem squarely makes a plea for the unwelcome child and its right to live. Roosevelt's noble four freedoms already cover Sir Dugald's objectives and should not be extended by travesty.

We are, etc.

Ian Donald
John M McBride
Wallace Barr
James Willocks

The Assistant Editor of the *BMJ*, Dr SP Lock, wrote back suggesting many changes and Ian replied to him in characteristic vein.

Dr S P Lock
Assistant Editor
British Medical Journal
BMA House
Tavistock Square
LONDON WC1

Dear Dr Lock

Freedom to Destroy Life

Thank you for your letter of the 29th of November.
Your legal adviser clearly recommends the removal of
most of the teeth of our letter, incisors, canines and all,
leaving only one or two wisdom teeth. We have no
interest in subscribing our names to a dull letter and
therefore accept your rejection in toto.

Yours sincerely

Ian Donald.

This was Ian's first brush with the medical (and political)
establishment. The Home Secretary, the formidable Roy Jenkins,
was a keen reformer, abolishing theatre censorship, legalising
homosexuality and supporting the Abortion Act. Subsequent
disputes cost Ian dearly and we are certain that the denial of
some public honours due to him was because he spoke his mind
and was never 'politically correct'.

Despite their debates on abortion and related topics, Ian
Donald and Sir Dugald Baird remained on friendly personal
terms. Ian was well aware of Sir Dugald's genuine greatness and
sincerity. Baird, in his career in Glasgow in the 1930s, was a
splendid practical obstetrician and coped with untold numbers
of crises. One of these was when the young Hector MacLennan

saw something unusual after a forceps delivery he had performed and could only stammer "send for B–Baird! It's b–bowel!!". Baird came and sorted it out.

In 1937, he was appointed Regius Professor in Aberdeen was already famous for community work, stemming from the Rowett Institute, run by John Boyd-Orr, nutritionist and health campaigner (later, as Lord Boyd-Orr of Brechin, he was Chancellor of the University of Glasgow) who was awarded the Nobel Prize for Peace in 1949 in recognition of his work towards alleviating world hunger.

Sir Dugald Baird's influence has been enormous and many university chairs have been filled by his pupils. Similarly, Ian Donald's influence was worldwide when ultrasound was accepted as the 'new diagnostic science' which it was.

To sum up the relationship between Baird and Donald, Baird was a rational Roundhead and Donald was a charismatic and somewhat quixotic Cavalier. Both were great men.

When Ian Donald gave his Charter Day Lecture at the National Maternity Hospital, Dublin, in 1972, the Abortion Act was firmly, but recently, on the Statute Book and he reflected on its implications in characteristic incisive terms.

> The passage of the Abortion Act in 1967 in the UK is only a signpost in a changing world, a result more than a cause. I think it is necessary for all of us to take stock on the effect on ourselves as clinicians who find ourselves willy-nilly at the hub of ethical decisions. The professional status of the gynaecologist is under threat and if we cannot embrace the philosophy and exercise the judgement which that entails then we have no right to claim a status much above that of a plumber or technician. We already have in the United Kingdom a profession divided and bewildered for lack of staunch and enduring principles. Younger recruits to future gynaecology may find themselves discriminated against in places where the clinical workload is heavy and involves a high incidence of therapeutic abortion.

The gynaecologist of today is at greater hazard from refusing to carry out an abortion than from doing one on even the most frivolous pretext. The future of gynaecology has to reckon with a new morality which must be recognised. As Abraham Lincoln stated, 'The dogmas of the quiet past are inadequate to the stormy present'. The gynaecologist can hardly avoid involvement, although at the end of his curriculum he may know more about steroid metabolism than about the deeper and more meaningful aspect of human thought and behaviour. The pressure groups of today are of course plausible and the materialisation of their humanist philosophy is rampant. I find refreshment in St. Paul's denunciation in his letter to the Ephesians, 'For we wrestle not with flesh and blood but against principalities and powers, against the rulers of the darkness of this world, against wickedness in high places'.

We suspect that the "high places" he had in mind were Whitehall and BMA House.

Ian goes on to list fourteen important subjects in which the gynaecologist is likely to be involved. "Two subjects in particular are bound to be charged with emotion. One is concerned with the beginning of life and the other with its end in death, viz. abortion and euthanasia. The acceptance of the latter by the public is a logical and natural sequence of the other. The principle that life is expendable because of its nuisance value can hardly be confined within limits."

A discussion follows about all the other subjects – contraception for teenagers, sterilisation population control measures, antenatal diagnosis of fetal abnormality, non-resuscitation of the severely handicapped, problems of sex-linked abnormality, genetic counselling, artificial insemination of donated semen, selective human reproduction on eugenic grounds, in vitro human fertilisation, maintenance of human embryonic life in vitro and availability of human tissues, including fetal, for transplantation. It is a remarkably comprehensive list to be written thirty years ago and most of Ian's remarks are clear, prescient, and infused with human sympathy. Some are worth quoting. Here is an interesting story about a sincere and dedicated pioneer of legalised abortion, Alec Bourne.

In England, until the famous Rex v Bourne case in 1937, it was only lawful to terminate a pregnancy to save the life of the mother.

I knew Alec Bourne well in my youth. He taught me much about writing and he was a very scholarly man with a profound knowledge of Shakespeare. He deliberately and provocatively advised the Home Office in London that he was about to undertake an abortion of a young girl, I think aged fourteen, who had been raped, allegedly, by four guardsmen, who had invited her into a stable to see a horse without a tail. The inevitable pregnancy which followed was brought to his notice. It was decided to prosecute him and make a test case of it. Where Alec Bourne went wrong was that he prejudged the guilt of the guardsmen who had not yet been brought to trial and when the police came to him at St Mary's Hospital (and I have heard this story from his own lips) to ask him not to undertake the operation just yet because the girl was wanted as a witness for the prosecution, he had to announce to them that he had just done it. In this respect he was guilty of gross contempt of Court. It was, however, overlooked but the police had no option but to prosecute and the judge had no option but to pronounce him guilty. But a remarkable wangle was undertaken which only the English with their well-known capacity for twisting words and meaning, was utilised to secure his acquittal.

Mr Justice Macnaughton, I well remember, decided that this girl's life was really likely to be one without health if pregnancy were allowed to continue, and left without health was not even life at all, and therefore Alec Bourne was still within the meaning of the law. This established the precedent that abortion could be undertaken in the interests of the health of the mother, as well as of her life and, of course, health could then be stretched to include the psychological health as well and even that could be extended with a little ingenuity to include even the unhappiness of the girl who found herself with an unwelcome pregnancy.

The situation in Scotland had always been healthier as one might expect where the legal system is more rational and all that was necessary in defending a doctor was to establish that he had operated in good faith. Abortion was therefore likely not to arouse interest or comment provided no fees were charged and Aberdeen readily established its reputation for integrity in this respect.

The Abortion Bill introduced in Parliament and passed in 1967 was compassionate in intention and endeavoured to regularise the situation which was obviously one of some sophistry. Basically it was a simple Bill couched in straight English of unequivocal meaning and endeavoured to secure safeguards against abortion on demand and racketeering. That it would fail in its objectives was obvious to me and many others from the very first. In all this unhappy controversy there was a very noticeable tendency to ignore the possible rights of an unborn child who, after all, had most to lose.

While this is a generous tribute to a sincere pro-abortion pioneer, at the end the temperature is raised a little by uncompromising remarks about the rights of the unborn child and the likelihood that the Abortion Act, as written, would not be implemented.

On the next page, Ian defines his stand on the Abortion Act and one senses that, like the Biblical warhorse, he sniffs the battle from afar and says "Ah-ha!".

For two doctors to certify the need for the operation is a fatuous piece of legislation. It would be the same whether it was one, three or twenty. The Scandinavian idea of a tribunal would hardly be practicable in England where the findings would likely take so long to emerge that by the time they did the child would have already gone to school.

The British Parliament had neither the guts to press for abortion on demand, unlike the New York State legislature, nor to include Northern Ireland, although this may have been in deference to the supposed right of Stormont to self-government. Certainly Scotland was included in the legislation where clearly no need for legislation existed.

You will note that the so-called social clause in the British law only applies to the welfare of existing children in the family and yet the figures from the Department of Health and Social Security indicate that over one-third of legalised abortions undertaken are in the case of single women in whom, obviously, no existing children have to be considered.

There can be no doubt that the British public as a whole has largely accepted the legislation as indicating the right to abortion on demand and we are all subjected to the most extraordinary requests for termination on what can only be regarded as frivolous pretexts, for example, one woman who complained to us that by the time her wedding came off she would be too large to get into her wedding dress, or another whose mother complained to me that her daughter had just embarked upon a cookery course.

A matter which has surprised me very much is the readiness of so many of my gynaecological colleagues to supply an 'on-demand' service. I find it hard to believe that in their case it was only the fear of the law that had hitherto stayed their hand. Because of the very great differences in the readiness of gynaecologists throughout the United Kingdom to undertake abortion a streaming phenomenon has manifested itself. General practitioners quickly come to know which units will readily carry out abortion and which are likely to prove sticky. This, of course, diverts a greatly increased workload to the units who take a fairly free and easy view. Nevertheless, all of us find that it takes far longer to refuse an abortion than simply to give in and be done with it.

Because of the strict line which we in my own unit have taken, most of the requests come from doctors who are really seeking support in their view that the request for termination of pregnancy should be refused and, in fact, the number of requests has not risen at all over the years since the Act was passed and has remained fairly static at approximately only one a week. You may attribute our attitude as you like to moral rectitude or sheer bloody-mindedness but we are nevertheless unrepentant.

He goes on to report the opposition to his own point of view with some relish.

In my opposition I have had much abuse hurled at me personally. I have been called a hardliner, a hypocrite, a moral re-armer, a Roman Catholic and even a South African whose attitude towards women was not dissimilar to the attitude of the South African towards his natives. I should here point out that I was born in Cornwall and am not a Roman Catholic but a mere Episcopalian. Like many people who adhere to the Christian ethic, I think my own opposition is basically a distaste for being an accessory to trivialising the sexual relationship between a man and a woman, a very precious relationship, by getting rid of the inconvenience of its natural consequence.

After this there follows an account of Ian Donald's interest in unborn life.

> It is fascinating to watch the development to maturity of a new human being by some technique such as sonar to which I have devoted much of my research life.
>
> The observed miracle of healthy development is enhanced by recognising the cases in which it goes wrong, often recurrently so. It is particularly heartbreaking to witness the present day wanton policy in many centres of discarding into the bucket or incinerator so much healthy unborn life whose only fault is that it is unwanted. The world may be losing both its senses and its sensibility.

More than thirty years after these words were spoken, we recognise that they contain truth. The liberal crusade against traditional morality has not created Utopia. Sexual licence has left behind a gathering trail of damage and misery in sundered families, broken hearts, and the shedding of trust and security. Sexually transmitted diseases are increasing rapidly and abortion figures increase annually. In England alone, there are about 180,000 abortions each year, of which 35,000 are in teenagers. This has an effect on the practice of obstetrics and gynaecology. In 1972, Ian Donald finished his Dublin lecture as follows.

> I sometimes wonder what I would do if I were young again and on the threshold of my professional career. I wonder if I would have the guts or the philosophy to face the challenge and try to practice medicine as a gynaecologist that was both honest and honourable. Will the gynaecologist of tomorrow, I wonder, be able to withstand the humanist pressure groups that we may, in the words of a famous Anglican Collect, 'So pass through things temporal that we lose not the things that are eternal'. Or will we simply fall in with the new philosophy of expediency, to supply contraception without advice, abortion when contraception fails and a neutral attitude towards the vagaries of human behaviour? Would this be fulfilling the

traditional role of guide, philosopher and friend to our parents?

> I tell you naught for your comfort,
> Yea, naught for your desire
> Save that the sky grows darker yet
> And the sea rises higher."

"At the Receiving End"

Courage and faith

For most of his time in Glasgow, Ian Donald was beset with the consequences of heart disease. This was the result of rheumatic fever, which had affected him and his sister Margaret. In 1960, Margaret had a mitral valvotomy performed in Glasgow Royal Infirmary and died as a result. Open-heart surgery was at that time a much more risky affair than it is now. Ian Donald was aware of the risks because, while he worked in Hammersmith Hospital, Ian Aird, the Professor of Surgery, had done much to stimulate research in that field. WP Cleland performed the first operation, reported in the *British Medical Journal* in 1954 as "Assisted circulation by pump oxygenator during operative dilatation of the aortic valve". The pump oxygenator was devised by DG Melrose, medical cardiologist. Ian Donald later recorded that he was present in a very minor assisting capacity at this operation in 1953 when cardiopulmonary bypass was first used. Both Cleland and Melrose were his friends for many years and appear again in this chapter.

In the Autumn of 1961, when Ian Donald was in New York, he collapsed with atrial fibrillation. This event was associated with overwork, a typical instance of which was a trip to Stranraer in the extreme southwest of Scotland to demonstrate the vacuum extractor. JW had assisted him in this project and was anxious about the Professor's health as we set off about 5 p.m. to drive south. He became increasingly breathless and we were both glad when we returned to Glasgow at 1 a.m. The Professor was up and in theatre at 9 a.m. that morning.

In New York, Ian Donald had to make an important decision—should he stay there for treatment or go back home? The outcome was clear. He wanted to go back to the Western Infirmary, where he was attended by Alister Cameron, cardiologist, and George Smith, cardiac surgeon (later Professor of Surgery in Aberdeen). The experience of mitral valvotomy horrified Ian far more than he had expected, but he bore it all with courage and not without humour. Visiting him was always accompanied by an illegal sip of sherry for visitor and patient. He kept the bottle in the bedside locker and we think the ward sister turned a blind eye to it.

He made a good recovery and returned to full activity. But in 1969, eight years later, things deteriorated. He recorded, "It was with some apprehension that I faced a second thoracotomy, but the sheer misery of acute congestive cardiac failure drove me to change my mind, if only as an act of suicide. A large and very tender liver made getting in and out of a car purgatory and pulmonary congestion and hypertension had wrecked most

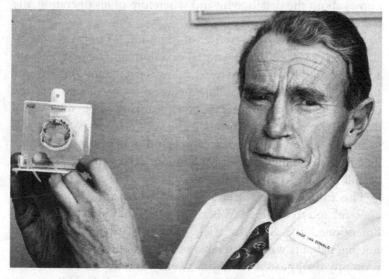

ID and old heart valve

nights' sleep over nearly two years. I repeatedly found myself reciting Keats' lines: 'Now more than ever seems it rich to die'."

This time he went back to Hammersmith Hospital and consulted Dr Melrose, physician, and Mr Cleland, surgeon. After cardiac catheterisation and angiocardiography, which had been undertaken under the full influence of warfarin, he had pelvic pain and urinary retention. Being alert to signs of residual bleeding, he felt a double mass in his pelvis – a haematoma. There was some doubt about this self-diagnosis, but the patient had the satisfaction of proving he was right by going over to a neighbouring hospital and getting an ultrasonogram taken, which demonstrated it well. His physician and surgeon took this in good part. Dr Melrose and Mr Cleland were united in their opinion that Ian required a cadaver aortic valve in place of his mitral valve, which was worthless.

Ian now set about acquiring all the information he could about the proposed operation, deciding that it was a good thing to be a doctor in these circumstances, even, as he put it, "a simple gynaecologist". He became convinced that the more a patient knows about the details, why and wherefore of his operation, the better.

He did not lose his sense of humour. "Two very merry anaesthetists visited me on several occasions and helped me with a little whisky I had tucked away in my locker. Soon our attitude showed signs of hilarity". The operation was a success, but the period spent in intensive care was traumatic. The removal of drains was particularly painful. "The sound of one's own voice yelling in acute pain is a demeaning and unnerving experience. The torture chambers of history and indeed of the present must be full of such harrowing incidents."

The attitude of the attendant staff, medical and nursing, was cheerful and this helped. When Ian developed pressure sores, he "mentioned the Scottish trick of using a sheepskin rug for nursing patients with vulnerable pressure points and my surgeon promptly disappeared for about twenty minutes and came back with one. He said he had been to Australia and shot it".

Being of a susceptible nature, Ian Donald soon found himself adoring all his nurses, getting out of bed to tease them rather than because of any belief in early ambulation. The attitude of the staff was not one of caution but of almost reckless encouragement to do anything he chose and to live life to his fullest capacity. This was in complete accordance with the personality of their patient. He recorded, "Three and a half weeks after my operation I took my leave and started on a course of convalescence which proved so strenuous, including the launching and commissioning of a small cruiser yacht on the south coast of England that I returned to my own department for a rest". He was back at work within nine weeks and a surgical colleague persuaded him to commit to writing his memory of his ordeal. A paper called "At the receiving end – a doctor's personal recollections of cardiac-valve replacement", appeared anonymously in *The Lancet* on 22nd November 1969.

The good effects of this operation lasted almost six years, but cardiac deterioration set in following an attack of subacute bacterial endocarditis. His Glasgow physician told him he could not expect to last out until retirement at the end of the current academic year without something being done and he was referred again to Hammersmith Hospital, where this view was confirmed. He needed no convincing to accept the replacement of his mitral homograft valve (a pig's mitral valve), which had served longer than most. Ian Donald later wrote, "My surgeon was very frank with me and, sitting on my bed, very patiently acquainted me with the odds". But the operation was very successful. The worn-out mitral homograft was excised and the largest and latest pattern of Starr Edwards plastic valve was inserted, partly because of the sheer size of the hole that had to be plugged and, as the surgeon explained, he did not wish to operate again. Ian thought that the speed of his recovery was "fantastic" and to be attributed to the ever increasingly meticulous attention to detail, including all the technical and back-up services "which are only available in so-called centres of excellence, a term very richly deserved". However, no major cardiac operation can be without pain. Ian admitted,

> I would be a liar if I did not straight away admit that this defies description. For the first week after operation the sensory system is presumably swamped by the sheer magnitude of the pain. After the first week there is more room for discrimination and I found pain and time, especially at night, to be poor companions.
>
> I often reflected that the pain must be akin to that of crucifixion minus the inevitable dislocation of the shoulders and the fearful injuries to hands and feet, and I am not ashamed to admit the great help vouchsafed to me by such thinking.
>
> The throughput of cases in this cardiothoracic unit staggered me. Commonly, two cases such as mine were done in a day. There were lots of us having this kind of surgery and there developed among us all a wondrous fellow feeling reminiscent of my days in the Royal Air Force during the war. We came from all walks of life and all sorts of background, from a great number of different places. They knew that I was a doctor and a professor of gynaecology, but did not hold that against me.
>
> I would like to acknowledge the unobtrusive but highly efficient chaplaincy service. I well remember the halflight of dawn at a time when I was in considerable pain when the padre swiftly and unobtrusively converted my bed table into an altar complete with candles. The nurse had asked me if I minded being joined by other patients to which, of course, I agreed readily. I was in fact joined by 'all of them' who themselves were waiting for his operation. Never had I thought the English of Cranmer more beautiful and after the padre had unobtrusively left, we stayed chatting together as dawn broke and another patient brought us cups of tea.

As in my own hospital, there were no apparent rules and it was natural that my wife should bath me; stitches, pacemaker and all. The atmosphere of sanity and freedom permeated the whole ward and it was a pleasure to get to know the wives of some of my companions.

The final encouragement came from my surgeon who, when bidding me farewell, said he had one instruction. My spirits sank as I anticipated some form of restriction. On the contrary, the instruction was not to be content with sailing my little twenty-six-foot sloop up and down the west coast of Scotland but to cover the entire west coast of the United Kingdom and, furthermore, not to leave the heavy anchor work to my all-too-willing wife.

Those who had read the account of Ian Donald's second operation in 1969 may have been struck by the thought that he was wearing his heart upon his sleeve, as evidenced by displaying the ultrasonic photographs of his haematoma in lectures. The same people were astonished when, in the account of his third operation published in 1976, he was not only wearing his heart upon his sleeve but had displayed it to view in glorious technicolour photographs which he used in subsequent lectures. They may have also been disgusted by the "gory details" of psychiatric decompensation and faecal impaction, which are given in this account. Ian Donald was not a man for beating about the bush. He recounted things as he saw them, and at the same time sought publicity. He got it.

Despite his egocentricity, his Christian devotion was sincere and increased with advancing age, as it does with many. Ian's religious feelings were displayed in a rather bizarre Good Friday broadcast on the BBC.

In it, he concentrated on the anatomy and pathology of the Crucifixion, drawing a comparison with the pain associated with modern cardiac surgery. He felt he had endured the sufferings of Christ in his own body:

"See from his head, his hands, his feet
Sorrow and blood flow mingled down."

Ian Donald was President of the Scottish Branch of the Order
of Christian Unity, an ecumenical society which sought to bring
together Christians of all denominations to discuss moral issues
of the day. At a meeting in Edinburgh in 1977, the year after his
third cardiac operation, he addressed the society on the theme
"Does Christianity Help?". He began,

"The title which was given me for this talk was "Does
Christianity Help?". I think I would prefer "Does Christ
Help?". I refer particularly to a person rather than a system.

Being a doctor

Does belief in Christ help in one's clinical practice and
decision making? It may surprise you to learn that although
it may make decisions clear enough, in practice it may
provide endless trouble and problems for the believer. In
this respect, gynaecology is a particularly vulnerable branch
of medicine. In gynaecology it is easy enough to know
what is right but this may involve swimming against the
tide today.

I need only mention the subject of abortion without a
proper and honest reason. As you may know, I have
consistently campaigned against the wanton liberal policy
of abortion on demand or request, however you like to
phrase it. Like so many of my profession I feel that to carry
out any surgical procedure on a patient without a good
reason is highly unethical; and when that operation involves
the sacrifice and destruction of the life of another it is
indefensible to regard the matter as trivial.

Not an absolutist

I don't think that one can or should be an absolutist in the
matter of abortion. A value judgement, that hateful phrase,

must not be shirked. One's Christian outlook inevitably influences that judgement. Would Christ Himself, who did so much to heal others of their afflictions, have supplied abortion on demand? I think not. Where the mother's health or life is at severe hazard there is really no problem, since one might lose both. These cases are now rare thanks to the advances in medical care which makes it possible to save both; in fact in many cases of severe heart disease in the mother it is often possible to get her through her pregnancy and delivery fitter than she was before.

The problem really comes when confronted with serious fetal abnormality, the likelihood of which can now be so often foreseen, thanks to modern diagnostic aids. At what point does one decide whether an unborn child has got the expectation of a life worth living, bearing in mind that to conserve such a pregnancy may increase the hazards to the mother meanwhile?

There are all degrees of abnormality and handicap from the very severe which may be incompatible with eventual survival to genetic or congenital disorders which, though distressing particularly to the parents, may still leave the baby with the chance of a happy and useful life. Sometimes such diseases are treatable after birth but more often they are not. Unfortunately this applies particularly to disorders associated with mental handicap – surely every pregnant woman's greatest dread.

Christian compassion

The destruction of perfectly healthy unborn life in healthy women because of the great nuisance value foreseen, rightly or more usually wrongly, and as a means of long-stop contraception, because of failure or neglect, is something which one could never regard as God's work. Here one is at once in conflict with current opinion in today's changed world. How difficult for a Catholic now, or anyone with religious belief, to get on in gynaecology where these bristling problems abound.

At the other end of life comes euthanasia. We all must die. Even Lazarus must have died a second time after being given a second innings. There should of course be no need to consider euthanasia as a matter of policy. All that is needed is tender loving care, the relief of pain by the judicious use of drugs which do not depersonalise the patient and allowing them to slip away with dignity and in peace. Nearly all the deaths in my department were due to advanced cancer. Wanton resuscitation by means which can only be called extraordinary such as cardiac massage would be neither Christian nor kind. I know that the interval between brain death and final death may be almost indefinitely prolonged nowadays. But I have found the problem in my own practice more imagined than real.

Cardiopulmonary death is nothing. I have been through that myself more than once. I recall the words of the poem:

> Existence is more than the taking of breath
> There's more to the gift than the giving
> And dying is more than the moment of death
> And life's more than a matter of living.

To be a pilgrim

Remember John Bunyan's verse:

> "Who so beset him round with dismal stories,
> Do but themselves confound, his strength the more is,
> Then fancies flee away, I'll care not what men say,
> I'll labour night and day to be a pilgrim."

The miracle of the world being transformed in a ministry of only three years and culminating in crucifixion is miracle indeed as Gamaliel well recognised. We ourselves recognise the hand of redemption in the Resurrection by which God proved His love for us. I myself have found it hard to understand why God should show such love for us because we are not very lovable. Well might we say 'Lord, I am not worthy that thou shouldst come under my roof'.

I love the motto of my University of Glasgow – *Via, Veritas, Vita*. The way, the truth and the life. And so it is very meet right and our bounden duty that we should at all times and in all places give thanks to Thee, Father almighty and everlasting God. Note that: 'At all times and in all places'.

Prayer

The habit of daily prayer preferably morning as well as evening and throughout one's day whether spent as doctor or labourer is easily acquired and should be maintained however poor its quality from time to time. Even in my old age I see, now and again, something fresh and comprehending in the Lord's prayer, for example, "Give us this day our daily bread". Note "this day" not tomorrow, or the next or when we fall on hard times or retire or become redundant.

My favourite morning prayer is the famous one which starts 'Prevent[1] us O Lord, in all our doings with thy most gracious favour, and further us with thy continual help; that in all our works, begun continued and ended in thee, we may glorify thy holy name'. I have taught myself the habit, however poor and automatic of giving thanks at the end of each care journey for example, thanks for not having hurt anybody.

And then the climax of one's devotions, the Eucharist itself. Here I speak as an Episcopalian – a Piscie – and do

---

1 'Prevent' means 'go before' – not 'stop'

not expect everyone to feel as I do. Remember, 'In my house are many mansions'.

Years ago, a medical student with me, who went down with tuberculosis, drew my attention to the prayer of humble access: 'We do not presume to come to this thy Holy Table' ... and which goes on to finish with that wonderful sentence 'that we may ever more dwell in Him and He in us'.

To all of us Christ said, "When I am lifted up I will draw all men unto Me". If only I could give back half as much as has been given to me. This leads me to conclude by quoting from my favourite hymn, 'When I survey the wondrous Cross'. The last verse of which reads:

'Were the whole realm of nature mine
That were an offering far too small
Love so amazing, so divine
Demands my life, my soul, my all".

Ethical issues concerned Ian Donald until the end of his life. In his Simpson Oration, delivered at the invitation of the Royal College of Obstetricians and Gynaecologists on 1st October 1976, just after he retired, he discussed the subject of "Superfecundity".

In it he said, "Human reproduction is no longer a matter that can be left to chance. That the sheer fear of an unwelcome pregnancy should influence, even dominate, the lives of so many healthy women is to emphasise the inherent vulnerability of their sex, which no liberation movement can properly neutralise without penalty since no form of contraception exists that does not exact its particular price. Abortion, as a longstop method of contraception, trivialises not only sex but life itself. Contraceptive techniques and family planning, in so far as they make possible responsible parenthood, are among the great boons of our age but in so far as they facilitate licence and abuse their effect can be socially disruptive".

Donald was always afraid that the gynaecologist would face increasing difficulties and in a prophetic paragraph he said, "Gynaecology is the first fully clinical branch of medicine to be subjected to political or lay pressure. It may not be the last; and the recently worsening image of the medical practitioner, both in the UK and USA, may bring forces to bear on our profession that I fear. Obviously geriatric medicine is next on the list and genetics and psychiatry are not far behind, as life becomes more expensive in one sense and cheaper in another".

He went on to describe a method he had devised recently: a non-pharmaceutical, non-invasive method of detecting the time of ovulation by a thermistor device that the woman could use herself. Unfortunately, it was too late in the day for him to introduce this into clinical practice, for he was already retired and in failing health. JW remembers Ian on a visit to Glasgow in 1983 asking him to line up some patients on whom he could try this technique, with their permission. On arrival at hospital he said, "It's all right. The apparatus is already sterilised. I boiled it up in the hotel kettle this morning!". Unfortunately, the hotel kettle had damaged the apparatus and the experiment had to be abandoned.

Nonetheless, he received recognition for his work on early pregnancy, fetal life and future interest in atraumatic contraception from the highest authority. He was invited to an audience with Pope John Paul II at the Vatican in 1979. Before that, Ian had been invited to Milan. Alix Donald recounts, "he showed a real-time film of an eight-to-nine-week fetus, perfectly formed, with all four limbs moving energetically, which infuriated a lot of Italian women in the audience who hoped for an abortion law in Italy. The film seemed to make it unthinkable. Ian was hurried out by the back door in case of trouble". The Pope was, of course, delighted and received Ian very kindly in Rome, speaking excellent English. He took Ian's research seriously, and a Cardinal in attendance carried some of Ian's reprints on ultrasound and other matters on a tray. Afterwards, Ian recounted, "You know, His Holiness talked to me for more than half-an-hour". On hearing this, WB responded, "I have never heard of anyone getting away from Ian Donald in under half-an-hour". He was truly a man of irrepressible spirit.

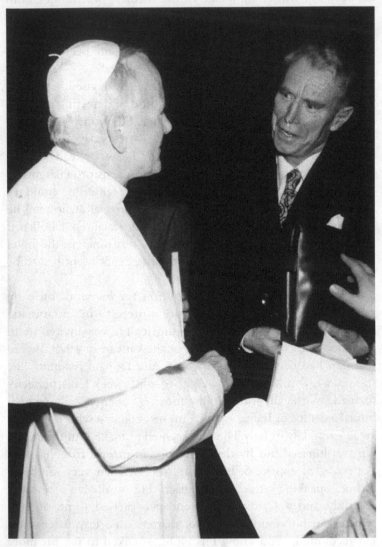

The Pope and ID

"The Evening Cometh"

International Fame, continued Battle with Illness and Home
Happiness in Retirement

On the day of Ian Donald's retirement, 1st October 1976, the
Royal College of Obstetricians and Gynaecologists, under the
presidency of Sir John Dewhurst, convened a celebratory
meeting in Glasgow, on which occasion Ian delivered the James
Young Simpson Oration, quotations from which have already
been given. It was a splendid occasion in the University, but those
who knew him best were a bit anxious about his ability to deliver
this long lecture. But despite breathing difficulties, he made it. Ian
Donald frequently said, "Retirement is hateful", but, despite
failing health, there were enjoyable features which brought him
into the public eye which was always a tonic for him.

Less than a month after his retirement he gave an interview to
Jean Donald (no relation), a well-known journalist on the
Glasgow Herald, which appeared in the newspaper on 27th
October 1976 under the title "Gentle Doctor in a World of
Women". His friends were slightly amused by this title, for
although he was basically gentle and kind he was also stimulating,
controversial and combative. This was recognised at the
beginning of the article.

Ian Donald is a man who cares about women and babies
but is the most outspoken anti-abortion doctor in Scotland.
The readiness to express his feelings of this subject has
tended to overshadow the major accomplishments of this
elegant, quietly spoken man in improving maternity care
for women all over the world. His pioneering work in the
introduction of ultrasonic methods of investigation in

obstetrics and gynaecology has saved the lives of hundreds of babies.

He said "I've seen a baby's heart beating in its mother's womb at a few weeks old. To me they are human beings and have a right to live. It's an everyday miracle and if preserving a few lives means that some people hate my guts I really don't care. I retired officially four weeks ago but I haven't stopped working since".

He has been married for almost forty years to Alix, a serenely pretty French South African. He said, "The three most important days in my life have been my wedding day; the day I went to a Glasgow engineering firm and proved that their ultrasonic equipment could be extended for use in medicine; and the day twelve years ago when the Queen Mother opened my hospital".

Ian Donald not only chose the location of the Queen Mother's. He chose the name. "I wasn't going to be upstaged. We already had the Royal Maternity Hospital in Glasgow, so I wrote to the Queen Mother and, much to everyone's surprise, she offered to open the hospital".

The Donalds' sitting room in his terraced home in the west end of Glasgow is dominated by a grand piano, the heart of family life when the girls were young. The eldest is now 36, youngest 17. The piano will obviously be in use tomorrow after the wedding of Margaret, the youngest daughter. "I know she's very young, but her boyfriend is very nice, a policeman". In a home dominated by women, Ian Donald has still managed to keep up some very individual pursuits – sailing (he has built three boats with his own hands) and painting.

But the women in his life have obviously strengthened his intentions of improving conditions in maternity hospitals. One may not agree with many of Professor Donald's sentiments but no one could doubt the sincerity of his beliefs.

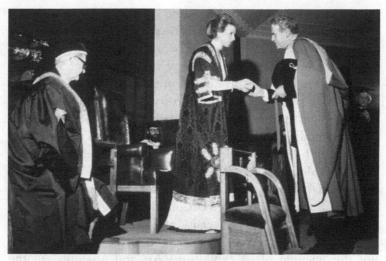

ID and Princess Anne, receiving the Degree DSc London

We have included the above extracts from the *Glasgow Herald* article because to us they ring true and skilfully give a picture of his character.

Despite being 'politically incorrect' at home, Ian Donald received recognition and honours. He was appointed CBE in 1973 and received the order of the Yugoslav Banner with gold star in 1982 for his work in developing an ultrasonic diagnostic centre in Zagreb. He received honorary DSc degrees from London (1981) and Glasgow (1983). He was awarded by the RCOG its highest honour, the Eardley Holland gold medal, the Blair Bell gold medal of the Royal Society of Medicine and Victor Bonney Prize of the Royal College of Surgeons of England. The Royal College of Radiologists made him an Honorary Fellow and awarded him the MacKenzie Davidson Medal. Other distinctions were FCOG (South Africa), honorary FACOG (USA), honorary FRCOG and honorary FRCP (Glasgow). He relished these distinctions to the full and enjoyed the associated ceremonial. But his health on these occasions sometimes caused anxiety. A striking example was the award of Honorary DSc at Glasgow on the University Commemoration

Day on Wednesday 15th June 1983. The university administrators were in a panic lest he should collapse in the vast crowded Bute Hall on this grand occasion. Should they have an ambulance in waiting? Should they have a team of stretcher-bearers in the hall ready to carry him out? We assured them that all would be well, but they looked very doubtful. In fact, despite showing signs of incipient cardiac failure at the beginning, Ian emerged smiling and enjoyed the whole thing. The university authorities should have been more relaxed, for a rehearsal of this event had already taken place on 14th April. 1983 marked the bicentennial of the death of William Hunter, the famous eighteenth century obstetrician, anatomist, art collector and great benefactor of the University of Glasgow.

A whole series of events had been arranged and one of them was the opening of an exhibition "Art and Anatomy" in the Hunterian Art Gallery, celebrating *Hunter's Anatomy of the Human Gravid Uterus*, a magnificently illustrated book and a great contribution to research. For the first time the original drawings of this work by Jan van Rymsdyk were on view. Ian Donald was invited to open the exhibition. He seemed scarcely able to breathe as he walked very slowly towards the small rostrum and had to be helped on to it. He then talked for about half-an-hour on "The Anatomy of the Dead", paying tribute to Hunter, and "The Anatomy of the Living," which was, of course, ultrasound. Theatrical solo performances stimulated him and he came off the rostrum much better.

Despite bad health, he continued to make foreign trips, lecturing and demonstrating, in his retirement. When he retired he was offered a consultancy with Nuclear Enterprises Ltd of Edinburgh, who specialised in making ultrasonic equipment and played an active part there until in 1981 he "emigrated to Essex".

The place that Ian and Alix chose was Paglesham on the Essex estuary, between the River Roach and the River Crouch, among a network of small rivers. To the east is Foulness Island, which is marked as a 'danger area'. The area is noted for yachting and boatbuilding and also for its oyster beds. The River Crouch is the headquarters of the Royal Corinthian Yacht Club. It is not difficult to see why the Donalds chose Paglesham for their retirement. They were happy there.

But health problems increased. Even before his second heart operation in 1969, Ian wrote to WB from Hammersmith Hospital, "As you know, I greatly fear the onset of incompetence, both clinical and scientific, which is part of the natural ageing process and the Western Infirmary has furnished, even in my own time, enough instances to put me almost obsessively on guard. Only about seven years to go, if I last that long, but I would like to keep all guns firing to the last". Fortunately the two valve replacements, in 1969 and 1976, saved his life and kept the guns firing remarkably well. However, the beneficial effects of surgery could not last forever.

We saw Ian and Alix last in Glasgow in May 1986 when they stopped on their return journey from Orkney where they had been visiting their daughter Christina. Despite their difficulties their courage and humour was evident as usual, but after that things began to go wrong.

On 23rd December 1986, Ian wrote to WB that the year had been disastrous with ill health involving "not only me but poor Alix as well. Admittedly my own cardiac nonsense and the prospect of widowhood so imminent were cause enough but I guess she had just about had all she could bear". On top of the strain, Alix had a spinal operation on the upper lumbar vertebrae, which was successful in ridding her of her limp, but not the sensory symptoms. Then she developed acute abdominal pain with all the signs of acute appendicitis. The surgeon correctly diagnosed a perforated diverticulosis. The operation included a temporary colostomy, which she accepted very courageously. A few months later she went for a follow-up X-ray and she perforated on receiving the colonic washout.

A massive operation followed, where the surgeon removed a large part of the descending colon, oversewed each diverticulum in the remainder and anastomosed the colon with the rectum, thus getting rid of the colostomy. Alix was delighted with the

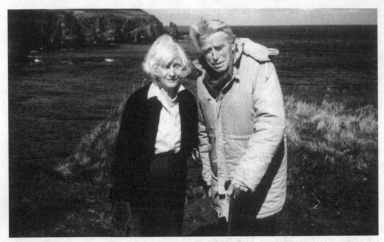

Ian and Alex in Orkney 1987

result and made a good recovery. Throughout her life, Alix has displayed love and courage in full measure and we should like to pay tribute to her here. In this letter, Ian went on to describe his own problems.

I am living on enormous doses of diuretics which keep me running day and night but at least it has got rid of my ascites and oedema; but the nights particularly are nightmarish, fighting for breath with my pulmonary fibrosis due to mitral back pressure. This induces a sort of panic breathing, having to fight for breath in spite of four or five pillows. I am now dependent on oxygen cylinders which are too heavy for me to lift and I have lost so much weight that you would hardly recognise me, now down to ten stone four pounds, faded but neither grey nor bald. On top of this I have cardiomegaly and atrial fibrillation and live on warfarin, which is checked by the haematologists in Southend. Nevertheless, I bleed at a touch and the backs of my hands are disfigured with echymoses, arms too. My electrolytes are all to blazes and cramp and gout, with a twice normal uric acid level which requires allopurinol to control it, complete the sorry picture.

I am too breathless to sail, have had to sell Chariessa and buy a Cornish Coble in its place but, even so, I cannot manage the six-metre rise and fall in tide even on a concrete slipway and my exercise tolerance is down to about fifty metres on the flat and no talking either.

Tessa and Odd,[1] suddenly realised our plight. Now Odd is a fully fledged orthopod and Tessa has gone back into general practice where the pay is better than her ENT consultantship.

She phoned up after yet another spell in hospital where my wretched doctors will not let me die what with their drips and oxygen inhalational therapy on which I depend. The Coble, a wizard little performer, sits in our garden on the off-chance that the sun might come once more and that I might yet sail again. Meanwhile an icy wind howls for days on end. Heathrow is too far, Gatwick little better and I long to come back to Scotland to see you all. Tessa phoned up last Easter and said she would come and fetch us if we did not take ship to Gothenburg where she would meet us. To the disapproval of my cardiologists, who regarded my condition as terminal, I got a ship from Harwich and arrived in a wheelchair. Tessa and Odd were there to meet us, oxygen cylinders and all, and she went into action, and I returned after five weeks to Southend in triumph minus the ascites and oedema. The journey to Hammersmith is too formidable and a superimposed fresh respiratory illness will close the chapter. Our happy days at QMH and WIG seem like another world and life. What fun we had. I will not trouble you again with all these disappointing details but you did ask for news. King Charles II apologised to his court for being such an unconscionable time a-dying! Same here! I hate being no damn use to man, woman, child, beast or devil.

With much love, Ian

---

1 His eldest daughter and son-in-law in Sweden.

Ian Donald's health deteriorated further and he died on Friday, 19th June 1987. The funeral took place in Saint Peter's Church, Paglesham on Saturday, 27th June 1987. The address was given by Father John Tracy, an old friend, who said, "I was familiar with Ian's characteristic style, and I am quite sure that the last thing he would want would be any undue solemnity in an address given in his memory".

He went on to describe Ian as "an outstanding obstetrician; an original and inventive medical brain; a brilliant lecturer; a formidable controversialist; a witty and humorous speaker; artist, musician, yachtsman. And more important than external activities, the inner personality. Ian was a man of great integrity of character. He held demanding principles and lived up to them; love of truth; honesty of judgement; outspokenness in comment and criticism; courage – conspicuous in his long struggle with ill health – and a profound respect for human dignity and the sanctity of life". This is a brief portrait that summarises the facts.

Another touching tribute was written by John MacVicar, who had, with Tom Brown and John Fleming, attended the funeral.

I stood beside Tom Brown at the graveside in Saint Peter's Church, Paglesham, as Ian Donald was buried. Little wonder that our thoughts went back over thirty years to the time when the three of us started to work together in 1956. All that was available then was a crude machine, which used ultrasound to detect flaws in metals and with it we were attempting to detect 'flaws' in women. Hours of continuous work often late at night became usual. Examination of countless patients and experiments with mechanical developments and picture display took up much of our time. Feelings of fatigue and frustration, despair and delusion, excitement and elation became well known to us. Recognition of the birth of a new science was slow. Personally, I might have given up the whole idea in the face of the current carping criticism but that was not for Ian Donald. He proved himself a man of vision who could see, despite all the criticism, the amazing potential which the new technique had. He pioneered something which as it developed was used worldwide and on which much of modern obstetric practice depends.

The title for this chapter, "The evening cometh" is taken from a famous prayer by Newman: "O Lord, support us all the day long of this troublous life, until the shades lengthen, and the evening cometh, and the busy world is hushed, the fever of life is over, and our work done. Then, Lord, in thy mercy, grant us safe lodging, a holy rest, and peace at last".

A memorial service was held in Glasgow University Chapel on 28th October, 1987. JW gave the commemorative address in which he said, "If you seek his memorial, look around you. In every maternity hospital you will see ultrasound in use. A great discovery by a great man.... I like to think that he had many glimpses of heaven before the end. 'My thoughts are more on the next world' he used to say in his latter days— although that did not prevent him from making trenchant and humorous comments on this world! And so he passed over— in the sure and certain hope of the resurrection and the life to come. Today, with his wonderful wife, Alix, happily present with us, and with members of his family, we remember him with affection and pride".

Ian Donald said that his chief ambition in life was to leave a name that would be remembered. Like the Roman poet Horace (another man who did not lack self-confidence), he could say "My work is done, a memorial more enduring than bronze. I shall not wholly die. I shall grow on and on in the praise of posterity".

We hope that this brief personal memoir will add a few more lines to that memorial.

Sources

London 1946–54

On the beginning of the NHS: Jennie Lee, My Life with Nye. Jonathan Cape Ltd; 1980.

On Hammersmith Hospital: Christopher C Booth, 'Half a century of science and technology at Hammersmith', in *Doctors in Science and Society*. The Memoir Club, *British Medical Journal*, 1987.

Appointment to the Glasgow Chair

Michael Moss, J Forbes Munro and Richard H Trainor, *University, City and State. The University of Glasgow since 1870.* Edinburgh University Press; 2000.

Sir Charles Illingworth, *University Statesman. The Story of Sir Hector Hetherington.* Glasgow: George Outram & Co Ltd; 1971. (Ian Donald's personal copy of this book, given to him by the author, is in our possession given to him by the author.) It contains a copy of a note from Ian to Sir Charles "You have done a great service, not only to his memory, but to the history of our University. I often consider that of all his Professors I have more reason than most to be grateful for his foresight and tenacity."

Andrew Hull, Hector's House; Sir Hector Hetherington and the academicization of Glasgow hospital medicine before the NHS. *Medical History* 2001;45:207–242.

Sharing enthusiasm

Ian Donald, *Practical Obstetric Problems*, 5th edition. London: Lloyd-Luke (Medical Books) Ltd, 1979.

The Western Infirmary
Loudon MacQueen and Archibald B Kerr, *The Western Infirmary 1874–1974*. Glasgow and London: John Horn Ltd; 1974.

The Queen Mother's Hospital
Ian Donald, 'The new Yorkhill maternity hospital'. *Scottish Medical Journal* 1961; 6:164.

The Queen Mother's Hospital, Glasgow, Clinical Reports 1964–71.

Science and Serendipity
Max F Perutz, 'I wish I'd made you angry earlier'. *Essays on Science, Scientists and Humanity* Oxford: Oxford University Press; 1998.

Wellcome Witnesses to Twentieth Century Medicine, Volume 5. *Looking at the Unborn: Historical aspects of obstetric ultrasound.* London: The Wellcome Trust; 2000.

Margaret B McNay and John EE Fleming, 'Forty years of obstetric ultrasound 1957–1997'. *Ultrasound in Medicine and Biology* 1999; 25 (1) 3–56.

List of papers by Ian Donald quoted in text:
Donald I. *British Journal of Non-Destructive Testing*, 1992

Donald I. (*BMJ*, 1977, 1, 555-560)

Donald I. Apologia: how and why medical sonar developed. *Annals of the Royal College of Surgeons of England* 1974; 54: 132–40.

Donald I. On launching a new diagnostic science. *American Journal of Obstetrics and Gynecology* 1969; 103: 609–28.

Donald I, Abdulla U. Placentography by sonar. *Journal of Obstetrics and Gynaecology of the British Commonwealth* 1968; 75: 993–1006.

Donald I, Brown TG. Demonstration of tissue interfaces within the body by ultrasonic echo-sounding. *British Journal of Radiology* 1961; 34: 539–46.

Donald I, MacVicar J, Brown TG. Investigation of abdominal masses by pulsed ultrasound. *Lancet*, 1958; i: 1188–95.

Donald I, MacVicar J, Willocks J. Sonar; a new diagnostic echo-sounding technique. Illustrative examples of ultrasonic echograms. The use of ultrasonic cephalometry. *Proceedings of the Royal Society of Medicine* 1962; 55: 637–40.

MacVicar J, Donald I. Sonar in the diagnosis of early pregnancy and its complications. *Journal of Obstetrics and Gynaecology of the British Commonwealth* 1963; 70: 389–95.

Willocks J, Donald I, Duggan TC, Day N. Fetal cephalometry by ultrasound. *Journal of Obstetrics and Gynaecology of the British Commonwealth* 1964; 71: 11–20.

Index

Printed in the United States
by Baker & Taylor Publisher Services